One Way or Another:
An A-Z of Real Birth Journeys

Compiled and edited by Rosemari Bainbridge

Dear Alice,

Thought I'd give Parcel Force
a miss, ha ha!

Can't wait to hear your
thoughts & hope you enjoy.

Rosie x

ISBN 9781686516115

2

This book is dedicated to those who help our little people arrive safely and with love.

Acknowledgements

Thank you, from the very bottom of my heart, to every mother and father who shared their birth story for this collection. Carving out time for such things in days filled with caring for and raising children alongside work, maintaining friendships and relationships, trying to be healthy, continuing those hobbies you enjoyed before you were required to change a nappy in the early hours with no wet wipes while administering Calpol is... tricky. Writing honestly, carefully, and passionately about a life-changing moment is undeniably brave. You're all superhumans.

Thank you, dearest reader, for buying this book. The money you spent will go to Wellbeing of Women – the UK's leading women's reproductive and gynaecological health charity – so that they can continue to fund life-changing and life-saving research for women and babies.[1] Once you've finished this book, I highly recommend visiting the charity's website – there you'll discover the true extent of their work's innovation, impact, and necessity.[2]

Thank you to my husband Alan for supporting, cheerleading, and occasionally reminding me that this project is actually worthwhile. And for designing the front cover, it looks ace.

---

[1] Wellbeing of Women is a registered charity. England & Wales: 239281. Scotland: SC042856.
[2] Wellbeing of Women (2019) *Wellbeing of Women* [Online]. Available at www.wellbeingofwomen.org.uk (Accessed August 2019).

Thank you to Jill Baker and Rosie Browning for being excited about this book from the very beginning and volunteering to proofread. My eyes had crossed.

Finally, thank you to my beautiful babies Phineas and Lincoln... Because your birth journeys really did change everything.

Editor's Note

Contributions to this volume arrived in a wide variety of forms – typed chronological recounts, audio recordings, handwritten notes, transcripts of conversations between friends… Some contributors wanted their work edited liberally (or even completely rewritten), while others did not. Some contributors are not native English speakers and none (as far as I'm aware) are professional writers.

As such, my editorial role has been threefold:

1) to respect all contributors' wishes and edit accordingly. All final edits have been approved by the authors;

2) to anonymise contributions. Any distinguishing details that might reveal the identity of an author to someone known to them (e.g. baby weight, weeks of gestation, place of delivery, etc.) have been included at the contributor's discretion;

3) to preserve each author's unique voice. These stories are so sensitive, so powerful, and so personal that I simply could not justify sacrificing authenticity for pedantic punctuation. To avoid interrupting a writer's flow with lengthy explanations of pregnancy and childbirth terminology, a glossary has been included at the end of the book.

I accept all responsibility for any glaring typographical errors. I will, however, assign blame to my wonderful children… They probably bashed the keyboard while I wasn't looking. Honest.

Contents

Introduction

In my family every birthday, every year is marked with *The Tale of How We Were Born*. Rushed ambulances to labour ward, the mopping of fevered brows, hurrying to push the baby out before the doctor arrived with those sharp bladed forceps… And descriptions of that horrendous, indescribable, and unthinkable *pain*. As a young girl I thought, "Why, in the name of all that is good, would anybody *ever* choose to put themselves through all that?!" I'd look down at my skinny body and think, "Nope, not worth it. Childbirth is for *chumps!*"

Then, in my early twenties, Mother Nature rang. And by "rang", I mean "soaked me in the overwhelming and inescapable desire to have a baby right then and there". There was no time for pregnancy. No time for planning. I needed a baby and I needed one *now*.

With my life's plot irreversibly twisted and my baby mania calming down just enough to book my IUS removal, the funnier moments from my family's birth stories slowly resurfaced – my father wearing a woolly jumper in theatre during a summer heatwave and passing clean out… My grandma worrying that her midwife was going to drown, so torrential the flood when her waters were broken… My mother-in-law going for a casual run when her contractions started, "Just to get things going!" As more family birthdays passed and the same stories were lovingly repeated and lovingly reheard, I began to notice moments when the speaker would fall quiet, gazing off into middle distance. Brief silences. The atmosphere would become heavy, light, poignant, flippant, reflective, and present, all at the same time. The emotions that childbirth induced were a complete and utter mystery to me… And I needed to understand.

After falling pregnant for the first time and a routine ultrasound scan confirmed that our baby was happy and healthy, I started preparing for labour. I simply had to know everything that there was to know about getting that baby out of my body and how that might feel. Yet while I could read ad nauseum about the physiological processes of childbirth, the emotional sides of the experience were only available in rather limited and extreme forms – from joyously breathing a baby out into the gentle waters of a brook to surprise deliveries in dirty supermarket toilets; from exhilarating freebirths on a best friend's couch to horrors of tearing so badly that two holes become one. Where were the *normal* birth stories?! How does a woman *really* feel during labour? And what could *I* realistically expect? Despite completing two hypnobirthing courses, attending more pregnancy yoga classes than I could shake my sofa-sized bump at, and suffering through a Parentcraft class where we got to see those dreaded forceps up close and personal, I was still none the wiser.

I've since birthed my two children and each experience could not have felt more different. While I'd been told by mums-of-many that every child's birth *is* different, *I* was welcoming two babies into the world within one year. As such, I made the totally unfounded assumption that I'd be exempt from this rule because my body was, to quote a heavily pregnant me, "Still in the birthing zone." (Pregnancy logic is a marvellous thing.)

Let me tell you about my first birth journey.

I was the expectant mother whose birth preferences were two and a half sides of A4 that my husband refused to laminate.

"But what if water from the birth pool splashes onto the paper and the midwife doesn't know that my 'contractions' should actually be called 'surges'?! And yes, of course this well-thought-through and painfully crafted document is called my 'Birth Preferences', not my 'Birth Plan'… Because things don't ever go to plan, do they? … What do you mean that nit-picking over semantics doesn't mean that deep down I'm still expecting these *preferences* to go 100%, unwaveringly, and perfectly according to *plan?!*"

Oh, cringe.

So, what did happen to my preferred, definitely-not-planned-but-definitely-planned water birth in a beautiful midwife-led unit with hypnobirthing tracks to help me ease out my baby under a canopy of twinkly lights? It became a post-term chemical induction in a consultant-led unit that led to three failed ventouse attempts, an episiotomy, repeated efforts to clip the baby's head to monitor his vital signs, a spinal block in preparation for forceps, the manual manoeuvring of baby while still in utero, and an eventual, final ventouse delivery before a postpartum haemorrhage.

When the consultant was elbow-deep in my vagina, rummaging around as if hunting for loose change under a sofa in his bid to stop my 11lb baby from piling out shoulder first, I laughed. Loudly. With tears gathering in the corners of my eyes. A wave of relief had washed over me, from the top of my head down to the tips of my toes. I was in (over? surrounding? squashing?!) safe hands (or one of them at least!)… And I was flying high! My first birth experience was the polar opposite of what I'd wanted and yet here I was, soaking up every moment, relishing every emotion that coursed through my (quite rapidly emptying) veins.

If I'm being truthful, I was a bit disappointed that I hadn't felt the physical sensation of baby crowning. I did push, obviously, but the spinal block prevented me from feeling the exact moment when I'd succeeded. But I do remember the emotional ride of that moment – laser-beam focus on the end goal, the sheer effort of pushing with all my muscles and might, gratitude that every single person in that operating theatre was monitoring, supporting, and wishing for our success, fear that my perineum would never survive all this argy bargy, excitement and anticipation that baby would soon be here, a genuine worry that maybe I'd be the one woman who quite simply could not birth her baby and that I'd be left pregnant forever…

As a result of this experience, I had two secret desires for birthing my second child – no induction, feel the push. This time, my birth preferences consisted of a single line: "Minimal interventions but do what you must so baby arrives safely". And all my wishes came true! A spontaneous labour that lasted the sum total of fifteen minutes with baby's head crowning on the sofa in Costa (apologies to anyone who was trying to enjoy their breakfast croissant that morning). No episiotomy, no pain relief, no interventions. And yet, even though this time I'd experienced my "perfect birth", I was left broken.

During labour, despite my very best efforts, a disconnect arose between my physical, mental, and emotional selves. Each cruel contraction felt like my entire body was being smashed against a brick wall. There was no respite as I was smashed again, and again, and again against that unforgiving metaphorical brick. The fear of birthing in hospital was so intense that (during what I now know was transition) I actually walked out. Right out. Straight through those double doors, I left the building. The rage when I'd staggered to freedom, only to be greeted by a cloud of smoke puffed out by the stressed and weary, was red raw and I screeched at their attempts to kill my unborn child. A switch then flicked – maybe it was *the baby* who was actually trying to kill *me*.

The resignation and hopelessness I felt as my husband tentatively placed his arm around my shoulder and guided me back inside the hospital were soul destroying. I was so vulnerable. I consumed another foul-tasting energy gel that my friend had so kindly gifted during those early contractions (they were the only things I could keep down) and contemplated lying down in the middle of reception and just… Disappearing. Maybe then this all-consuming emotional and physical pain would vanish and leave me in peace.

The shocking contrast between these two birth journeys will never leave me.

*

Eva Wiseman, writing in *The Guardian*, raised an important question: "We need stories about giving birth, in all their gore and glory. So why are we so slow in sharing them?"[3] While my family were (and still are) open and honest when regaling their birth tales, I fluctuate between feeling fearful and hesitant when sharing mine. Sometimes I want to talk about my labours but don't know if the other person wants to listen. If I am asked to share my story (which is surprisingly rare… Surely bringing two new humans into the

[3] Wiseman, E. (2018) 'Childbirth Stories are the Stuff of Life. We Should Share Them', *The Guardian*, 8 April [Online]. Available at https://www.theguardian.com/lifeandstyle/2018/apr/08/lets-give-our-childbirth-stories-a-big-push-share-eve-wiseman (Accessed April 2018).

world is a feat worth talking about?), where do I start? Which bits do I pick? How long do I have the floor? When speaking with pregnant or soon-to-be-pregnant friends, I don't want to build up hopes or scare them, and I can never be mindful enough of others' birth experiences before I detail my own… And how do I cope with that acute flash of fury I feel when I'm interrupted or (even worse) laughed at? Over the last five years I've fundraised for the charity Wellbeing of Women and, as part of this voluntary work, blogged about a whole range of lived experiences in this female body of mine… And yet I can't bring myself to share all the details about either of my births. Why such fear?

Wiseman suggests it's not just me who feels this way.

The culmination of all this thinking and pondering is this very book – a collection of twenty-six real birth journeys told by twenty-six real parents. Created in an attempt to conquer these widespread fears of sharing birth stories and to start a desperately needed and healthy conversation about women's healthcare. The "facts" of each labour are not the focus of each story. Instead, contributors recall the emotions that they experienced during labour and the effects of what took place. In short, they relive their birth journeys and how they felt, every step of the way.

This book has three main aims. The first is to provide a kaleidoscopic snapshot of the childbirth experience. Contributors boast an array of social, religious, economic, and cultural backgrounds, ages, routes to pregnancy, countries of birth, health conditions, and number of previous birth experiences. The variety of expectations, outcomes, and reactions is staggering and the scope of what "normal" childbirth can look and feel like is thrown into sharp relief.

The second aim is to allow parents to share their birth stories uninterrupted. No quips of, "It couldn't have been that bad!" or "My friend had that!" or "So you didn't manage without pain relief?"… Or, for the ultimate guilt trip, "At least you have a baby." For some contributors, this piece of writing is the first opportunity they've had to share their birth journey in full. For some, their contributions contain those "hidden" emotions, those "secret" feelings that they believe (for whatever reason) they shouldn't or aren't allowed to feel. Disclosing such internal monologue, unedited, parts of which you know will prove unpopular with your audience of complete strangers, parts of which you might now, in fact, regret or even be ashamed of, is a courageous act. These raw, sometimes primal emotions (even if short-lived) are valid and deserve to be heard, acknowledged, and understood in the tumultuous contexts in which they were felt. I ask for each birth journey to be approached with the open, empathetic, and non-judgemental mindset that it deserves.

The third and final aim is to begin forging a language of childbirth – not just to list chronological, physiological happenings, but to describe how labour feels, at every stage, in all manner of circumstances. During the 2017 International Women's Day Debate in the House of Commons, Sarah Olney MP spoke of childbirth as "probably the ultimate feminine achievement". I agree when she said that "[w]omen are often told not to make too much of a fuss about childbirth":

> Yes, we discuss the timing and order of events such as what we were doing when we went into labour and how long it took, but we have not really developed a language to talk about how it feels or how it makes us feel. We just do not have the words.

> Although the experience leaves a lasting imprint, it is never fully acknowledged. The memory of childbirth remains with us – unshakeable and unshareable, but never fully expressed. [4]

I want to shout from the top of the hospital that I didn't want to be in about what a huge achievement it is for a woman to give birth – whether the experience was loved, loathed, boring, underwhelming, overwhelming, thrilling, numbing, or any combination of these emotions and more. I want this book to lead the way in developing a language of childbirth in which we can all be fluent. I want to empower mothers and fathers to share their birth stories and to encourage others to listen to these stories without interruption or judgement. And if, in the meantime, we can raise some money for a charity that supports labouring women, their babies, and their families, then so much the better.

---

[4] *Sarah Olney on International Women's Day* (2017) YouTube video, added by Liberal Democrats [Online]. Available at https://www.youtube.com/watch?v=LHqAbgMS28c (Accessed April 2018).

Birth Journey A

Labour *technically* started on the Tuesday (two days before our due date and my second day of maternity leave) but I only know that because the midwives at the hospital could measure some contractions. I couldn't feel them; I was only getting checked because I'd had a little bleed whilst out on a boredom-reducing five-mile walk and I'd panicked. I drove myself to hospital to the assessment unit and fought an old lady for a parking space. She wanted to park because her daughter was in labour, but I'd got there first and shouted, "I think I might need it more, I might be in labour myself!" Madness! Anyway, they made me stay overnight, even though everything seemed otherwise normal, and I felt a total fraud.

In the morning, the consultants told me that they thought they should induce me. For some reason this really didn't sit well with me; it felt totally unnecessary. I reasoned with the doctor that there was otherwise nothing else wrong and the baby seemed healthy, so why move so quickly to induction? He suggested that the baby was already ready to come out, there was no real reason to continue the pregnancy further, and any additional time was simply an unnecessary risk. In hindsight, he was making perfect sense but I was seriously not on board. He spoke to his superior and we compromised that they would book me in for an induction in six days' time and I would have to be monitored more closely until then. I'm not entirely sure what made me feel so confident to ignore decent medical advice but, on this occasion, I'm glad to say that it was a good decision.

When I got home on Wednesday lunchtime, I sat on the sofa and, within about two hours, I could tell that we were actually on our way to having a baby… Although it did just feel like I had an achy back. I felt really calm… Like when you've been revising for an exam for a really long time and you're finally sitting at the table, ready to start writing. There's nothing else you can do – you know everything that you're going to know, you just need to get your pens in order and turn over the page… And I couldn't wait to get the results!

I called my husband to say he should finish up his work as I didn't think he'd be back in the next day but, to be honest, I felt like I had lots of time. I baked a couple of cakes (we were going out for dinner and I'd said we'd bring pudding), called my parents and told them not to expect anything as almost no babies are born on their due date, and then, when my husband got home, we went off to dinner… Packing the hospital bag in the car "just in case" since our friends live closer to the hospital than we do.

During dinner the contractions got stronger and by the end (around 22:00), they were strong enough to force me to concentrate (although they still weren't painful). We went home, now pretty convinced that things were kicking off, and sat on the bed wondering what to do. By 23:00(ish), I decided I needed the TENS machine; that really took the edge off the contractions' intensity. But pretty much as soon as I started using it, my waters broke *all over the duvet!* I didn't know what to do! Should I move or stay still to contain the mess?! Eventually, I ended up sitting on the toilet, laughing about how glad I was that hadn't happened an hour or two earlier in my friends' dining room!

Another hour passed and I was now having to breathe through the contractions. They were pretty strong and about three were coming every five minutes. We called the hospital. They asked if I could still speak, which I could (I could actually speak through the contractions right till the very end, so maybe not the best test?) and so was told that I was still a way off and should stay at home. I was unconvinced, however, as it really did feel like things were moving along. The NCT leader had told us that first-time mums are often fobbed off with this sort of excuse, so I disobeyed, we got in the car, and headed to the hospital.

After being assessed, we were sent up to the midwife-led unit where I wanted to give birth. The midwives were reluctant to check my dilation as I'd only been contracting for a few hours; once they check, you have to stay in the hospital and they were quite convinced that would mean a *loooooong* wait. This was at about 01:00, so they thought I should go home and rest, but I really didn't think I could leave; the short journey in had been pretty intense. So, I convinced them to check. They were, unfortunately, correct – I was only 2cm dilated, not even technically in labour. The midwife suggested that, despite my initial objections, some pain relief might help me get through the next few hours and take the edge off enough to let me relax and things progress. She said that a Meptid injection was "like five vodka cokes," which sounded ever-so-nice at that point… I had the injection (that itself was suspiciously painful!) and headed downstairs to wait it out.

After forty-five minutes or so of sitting on a bed listening to Rufus Wainwright and trying to nap, things definitely ramped up… I ended up back on the toilet, this time less amused. I had very strong contractions that felt a lot like needing the loo, but nothing was happening. I felt panicked because the sensation had changed so quickly – this felt very different and I wasn't sure it was supposed to feel this way. We didn't want to hassle the midwives again, but I told my husband that we had to; if I was going to feel like this for eight hours or more, then I definitely needed an epidural (despite being absolutely terrified of them).

The midwives came in and tried to convince me to lie down so they could check my dilation but I really was struggling to do so between the contractions that were now coming thick and fast. I finally managed and, much to the midwives' surprise, I was 8cm dilated! Baby was most definitely on the way!

After spending some time convincing me to put my trousers back on (I was so far beyond caring about my dignity but apparently it wasn't okay to be naked in the lift), they wheeled me out and back upstairs. The midwife who met us was the same lady who'd seen me earlier. She was lovely and completely understood (or seemed to) my outrageous claims that the room they were busy getting ready for me was absolutely unsuitable as it had no windows(!) So they kindly moved me to one *with* windows and started filling the water bath as the sun rose over Oxford.

The midwives talked me through some breathing, and I was much more receptive to their guidance than I had been to my husband's (much to his dismay!) The Meptid had, by now, mostly worn off and I was relying heavily on my TENS machine. That thing is amazing. I was afraid to take it off to get in the water as I wasn't sure I'd cope without it but, as soon as I stepped into the bath, everything felt much better. I've always loved a nice relaxing soak and that's exactly how it felt… Despite being naked in a strange room with a relative stranger staring at me!

I began pushing. To be honest, this is the only bit I remember being *actually* painful… Although maybe that's rose-tinted spectacles? My husband was in charge of the gas and air, which really helped me get through the pushing stage... But even with that, I felt that this was the only part of the whole process where my body was asking me to stop whatever was going on because it was all too painful. Still, it was intriguing at least – between flirting with the midwife (my husband always likes to tell that part of the story!) and pushing, I was able to reach down and feel my baby's head crowning. That might sound weird to some people, but I found it absolutely incredible – to feel something like that happening to yourself! Having pushed out the head, I felt euphoric! And was dismayed to learn that you then also have to push out the shoulders – urgh! But I did and, as the rest of my baby came out in a big gush of blood (also something I wasn't expecting), I was able to reach down into the water and pick her up into my arms... What a moment!

The baby was still attached to me as my husband confirmed that she was indeed a "she" and not a "he". The water was now a little on the grim side, so we were asked to step out the bath and move to the bed. I couldn't quite believe what they were asking me to do! I wasn't sure that I'd be able to, but it turns out that you can, in fact, walk with a baby attached to you between your legs by an umbilical cord! Probably one of the more surreal moments of the whole thing!

My husband cut the cord, the midwives panicked about ensuring the baby was wearing a hat (apparently of paramount importance!), and the placenta came out, thankfully intact. I barely felt that happening, again another unexpected thing... Maybe I was too busy cuddling my little baby? The midwives checked three times for tears; apparently babies don't come out that quickly without tearing, but I was unbelievably lucky and still in one piece. And then they left us alone as a family of three with some tea and toast so that we could watch the day begin around us over Oxford.

Afterwards, I reckoned that I'd been pushing for around twenty minutes, although my husband thinks it was closer to two hours. Labour was such a blur and all that mattered was that, at 07:22 on her due date, our beautiful baby was born. Happy, healthy, wrinkled, and 3.72kg. And the clever little monkey latched straight onto my boob and began feeding from me. I felt completely on top of the world! I hope I never forget that feeling.

That was two years ago and every time I think through what happened during those twenty-four hours, I realise how extremely lucky I was. I'd always felt oddly confident that I'd manage without pain relief and I feel like I was guided really sensitively towards having some that was appropriate and given at exactly the right time. I'd tried to stay as healthy as possible during pregnancy in order to give me the stamina required for labour but actually my labour was only about seven hours long (officially about six hours) and was smooth sailing compared to some. And whilst my recovery took longer and I felt a lot more bashed around than I'd anticipated, I was so lucky to be able to hold my baby immediately, not need any additional surgery, and to shower and feel relatively normal again just a few hours after giving birth.

Whilst I think having a calm and confident attitude before things began really helped me at home during the first stages of labour, I think the hospital staff were simply amazing at supporting me through the more difficult parts; however prepared you are and whatever's happening, it's the first time you're doing it and it can be a lot to deal with. Two factors I think benefited me were (1) understanding the biology behind all points in the process, and (2) distracting myself as much as possible during labour. Going out for dinner was brilliant and I'm grateful for my very understanding friends who thought it was exciting and not-at-all weird that I turned up, despite possibly being in labour. And listening to music was really good when things were a bit tougher.

My husband was also really supportive. He listened to my needs the whole time and did everything that I asked him to do. He told the staff exactly what I wanted and clarified my requests around pain relief when appropriate. He let me choose when we went to hospital and, when we called the midwife, allowed me to feel in control, even when he was actually organising everything around me. Sadly, the massages and breathing that we'd learnt in NCT classes weren't much use… During most of the process I just wanted to be left alone! But my husband understood this and still tried valiantly to make me feel comfortable; he tried every single time I decided that some massage or breathing technique might work *now*, before I decided a mere ten seconds later that it didn't!

And the midwives were amazing. The Spires Midwifery-Led Unit was an incredible place to give birth, so calm and quiet – you birth in a lovely room with a lovely view and lovely midwives to help you through. You see the same midwife as far as is realistically possible and mine even stayed past the end of her shift to get me to the finish line as we were so close. When midwives changed shifts, they introduced themselves, and when they changed back again, the original midwife came to see me and the baby. After the labour, they encouraged me to shower and to feel normal again as soon as possible (shockingly soon!) and talked me through all the things that I needed to know about how my body would recover. We had a private room with a private bathroom, they brought me tea and biscuits through the day and night, and my husband could stay all day (not just for visiting hours). They even let him come in at 06:00

the next morning when I was seriously done with no sleep and with not being able to put the baby down!

We're expecting another baby to arrive in a few months and I can only hope that we have a very similar birth story. There's a lot of pressure on this one to be as good as the first! But I'm very grateful that I only have good memories of my first birth, which makes going into all this again a lot easier than I can imagine it is for some mums.

Birth Journey B

I was 39 weeks pregnant and had been feeling unwell for a couple of days when my waters broke at the unearthly time of 02:00 on Monday. I can only describe this feeling as if I'd just wet myself! I woke my husband up and he rang the labour ward to see what we should do. They suggested we get checked out, so we jumped in the car and he drove us to the ward. I felt anxious but not scared… I was ready and wanted to get started as soon as possible!

On arrival, we were seen very quickly by a friendly midwife who checked me, the baby, and its heartbeat. She confirmed that my waters had, indeed, broken, but that it was probably going to be a while; I could stay if I wanted but was advised to go home, relax, and wait for contractions to become regular. I was booked in for an induction on the Tuesday morning in case nothing happened. We knew other couples who'd gone home and that this was a normal thing to do at this stage in the proceedings, so we both felt pretty calm… Although one such couple did wind up having their baby on their bathroom floor! We assumed this was a rarity though… So, home we went.

My husband got straight into bed to get some sleep, as we knew every minute of sleep would probably prove valuable. I lay on the sofa to try and sleep too, having not slept much that weekend. Mild contractions that felt like bad period pain came every half an hour or so… I'm not sure I got any sleep at all. This continued throughout the night and into the morning.

I'd been to pregnancy yoga and hypnobirthing classes, so I was trying to use some of the techniques I'd learnt to get things moving, such as bouncing on a birthing ball... This was the sight my husband came downstairs to at 07:00! However, the contractions weren't getting much more intense or closer together. We spent the day trying to keep active and encourage contractions to increase – took a couple of walks into our village, popped into Sainsbury's for some tea, stuck with the birthing ball... I drank plenty of raspberry leaf tea as apparently this is supposed to help. By around 21:30, contractions had increased in intensity, duration, and frequency (to around every six minutes). To me, the contractions felt pretty powerful – but, with this being my first child, I didn't really have any point of reference! We rang the maternity ward again but were told not to come in as the contractions were still not close enough.

This continued into Tuesday morning, with contraction strength, length, and number varying quite a bit. At no point did we feel we could go into hospital, based on what the midwives had said. We both went to bed but I didn't stay there for long as I couldn't sleep (not helped by my husband's snoring!) Back downstairs and back on my birthing ball!

Around 01:00, my contractions felt quite intense and were down to four and a half minutes apart, so I got my husband downstairs... Before they started to vary and weaken again. My husband had the idea of us both getting into bed and cuddling – to try to relax and release some more oxytocin. This made me feel much better; the tiredness and frustration caused by the slow speed of the labour were getting to me. Contractions were still coming every five or six minutes.

By 05:30, we were getting a little nervous as we didn't want the labour induced, if at all possible. We also didn't want to get stuck in rush-hour traffic, so decided to go to my parents' house, handily situated just a short walk from the hospital. We arrived there for 06:30, called the hospital, and were told to ring back at 07:30 if nothing had happened. With the stress of this impending deadline, my contractions fell further apart (although I did have a couple of painful ones).

We arrived at the hospital around 08:00 and received a private room in the maternity unit. I continued to use my birthing ball but, by now, my contractions had all but stopped. I resigned myself to the fact that I was going to be induced... This did disappoint me as it was not going to be the "natural birth" I'd wanted... But I was still ready to get going and felt up for the challenge ahead!

We were seen by another really friendly midwife who put us at ease. She examined me and said she'd try to get away with not giving me the pessary (otherwise we'd need to wait six hours before we could have the oxytocin drip). Instead, she gave me a stretch and sweep; it felt, to quote the midwife, like she was "rummaging in my handbag!"

After some entertainment from a puzzle book and more birth-ball bouncing while we waited for a free bed on labour ward, the oxytocin drip was started.

Commencing induction did not exactly go smoothly. For starters, the midwife could not get the cannula in. She tried on my right arm, but a blood bubble formed thanks to a long-standing varicose vein in my right hand. She was then unsuccessful with my left arm, so went to get the junior registrar. He wanted to use my right arm but my husband, having seen what had happened the first time, suggested he check my hand first... He decided to go for the left wrist. He also struggled... But finally succeeded. My husband later told me that I'd left quite a pool of blood on the floor but rightly decided that now was not the time to divulge! All these details may seem fairly irrelevant (I'm sure such things don't happen that often) but they might explain why I felt rather anxious and even further separated from the ideal picture that I'd painted in my birth plan.

Speaking of birth plans, we had been told that they rarely work out. In our case, that is certainly true. I'd wanted to manage using my breathing, and maybe some codeine, and then, when the pain became too intense, gas and air. Although I didn't particularly want a water birth, I didn't rule out using the pool to relax in as I'm partial to a nice bath! Thanks to the induction, this was no longer possible… But I did still hope to manage the pain as planned.

Once the drip was in, contractions soon became more frequent and intense. Almost immediately, it turned out that the contractions I'd had at home, the ones that I'd thought were quite intense, were really actually very mild!

It's difficult to recall how much time has passed when you're in that room, in that situation; my husband says it's like being in a completely different time zone with a completely different set of rules. It was probably a couple of hours before the pain became too intense to manage with just my breathing and I needed codeine. If I'm honest, I don't really know if the codeine did that much – maybe just took the edge off. Throughout the midwife was very encouraging and was already asking questions about skin-to-skin, who would cut the cord, and whether I wanted the injection to birth the placenta… Given the intensity of the contractions and the pain I was in, we assumed we were pretty far down the line!

Unfortunately, we were wrong. I wanted gas and air (badly!), so the midwife examined me. I was only 2cm dilated. My heart sank. I knew I needed to get to 10cm and, given all that I'd been through up to this point, began to feel rather desperate. To make matters worse, the midwife said I could not have gas and air until I was 4cm dilated; it could potentially slow the contractions down when we needed to speed them up. She also told me that she needed to ramp up the oxytocin drip… Considerably. With no gas and air, this was not going to be fun at all.

I went on for as long as I could. I knew I was going to need something, but the midwife was adamant that I tell her what I wanted to do; she wouldn't *suggest* anything. It seemed very early to go down the road of an epidural. We'd heard bad stories about Pethidine… I was sure I didn't want it… But, at this point, it seemed the only option. My husband asked if they could examine me one more time, just in case I was now 4cm dilated. Alas – I was 2.5cm. I remember crying. A lot. We decided to go for the Pethidine.

With hindsight, this was a big mistake. Pethidine is supposed to "take the edge off"… It just sent me crazy. I felt the pain as strongly as before but I was completely spaced out, as if uncontrollably drunk. I do remember seeing the fear in my husband's eyes though – he looked completely terrified. Apparently, I was in agony and the contractions were coming every minute with incredible intensity. There was little to no respite. I threw up a number of times, although my memory of this is sketchy at best.

Eventually, there was no alternative but to have the epidural. This turned out to be the best decision I could have made. I only wish I'd made it earlier. *Much* earlier! After the epidural, I felt quite calm. I could see my husband was very glad to have a break from the screaming and wailing, and the helplessness that he felt. The midwife was now able to ramp the oxytocin drip up to the max and all I felt were two dead legs! With this pain relief I went from 2.5cm to fully dilated incredibly quickly and, before long, I was ready to push. I actually quite enjoyed the pushing phase!

During the birth, the midwives were struggling to get a consistent read on the baby's heartbeat from the band across my stomach, so we had to get her head tagged with a monitor. They seemed a little worried – every time I had a contraction, the baby's heart rate kept dropping below the norm.

When the baby started crowning, I seemed to go through a number of pushes without much progress. A student midwife focussed entirely on coaching me through the birth, giving me a fantastic pep talk for the last push... Unfortunately, she hadn't quite cottoned on that we didn't know the sex of the baby and kept saying, "I can see her head!" But finally, eventually, a baby, who was indeed a daughter, was born. The umbilical cord was wrapped around her neck twice, which explained the heart rate issue, but she was born healthy and weighing 8lb 7oz. They gave her a quick wipe down and put her on my chest...

The sensation when she was born was like nothing else I'd ever felt. The overwhelming relief is indescribable – relief that she was okay, that I was okay, that it was finally over! Baby soon gave a little cough and started to cry. It all felt *incredible* – you just don't know love like that until you experience it yourself. It was the same for my husband. These emotions made every minute of what we'd been through well worth it.

... Delivering the placenta is quite the epilogue! I had an injection to help it come out; this normally happens within about ten minutes. Forty minutes later and nothing. The midwives were getting a little nervous, but I was beyond caring... I had my beautiful baby in my arms! I was still sporadically throwing up thanks to the Pethidine when a few more midwives entered the room and started speaking with a doctor about the placenta… Suddenly, I threw up and, as I did so, the placenta just shot straight out! No-one was watching, they were still talking quietly in the corner, formulating a plan of attack. I shouted, "Err, the placenta's here!" My husband had to have a look. Apparently, it's the weirdest thing he's ever seen in his life!

My husband was by my side throughout. Later he told me that he'd just felt so helpless and rather scared; I was making noises he'd never heard before! He was amazing though, providing a constant supply of water and damp flannels to help me through.

Given how it all panned out, there's only one thing we'd change, on reflection – get the epidural sooner. We found out afterwards that when you have an oxytocin drip, the induction pretty much comes hand in hand with an epidural or a C-section. The midwife was adamant that I told her what I wanted but, having never been through that experience before, the decision was a very difficult one to make. Next time (if there is a next time), I don't think I'll make the same mistake again!

Our daughter is now three months old and she has changed our lives immeasurably. Life with a baby is certainly hard work and produces many challenges… But, without a doubt, she means the whole world to us and has already given us more that we could ever dream of. Bring on the next however-many years!

Birth Journey C

On 17 June 1986 (my due date), I had a hospital antenatal appointment. I had quite a difficult pregnancy due to prolonged sickness, weight loss, and breakthrough bleeds, including one at 23 weeks, for which the treatment at that time was bed rest. The fact I had made it to full term was an achievement in itself for us!

I sat in the hospital cubicle in my underwear waiting to be seen. Unfortunately, I saw a different duty doctor every time. The doctor asked my due date and when I said, "Today," he proceeded to do, *"An internal examination"* (as he called it). Following this, I was horrified to see that his hand was covered in blood, as was the paper sheet protecting the couch I was lying on.

"Go home and pack your bag and bring it back to the hospital," he said. "You are having this baby today!"

I was in agony with tummy cramps and felt quite faint, and the thought of driving home was awful – but I had no choice. I did as I was told.

I collected my already-packed bag and came back to the hospital where I was duly booked on to the maternity ward. It was very quiet. There were a few new mums with tiny babies in clear fish-tank cribs lying next to their beds on the ward as I was taken through another ward to my bed. By this time, I had really severe cramps, but I was told that was normal and to let the nurses know when they became stronger and more regular. I was left alone like this for hours. My usband came to visit at teatime and stayed for an hour, then he was ent home.

By 01:00, the pain was severe, and I felt as though I needed to se the bathroom. I managed to get to the toilet cubicle unaided nd, as I sat down, felt the loss of quite a lot of blood. I pressed the mergency buzzer in the loo and about five minutes later a nursing ssistant appeared in the doorway. I told her what had had appened and she was not pleased with me at all. I remember her aying, "You are not the only lady on this ward, you know. Others re having babies too!" I was horrified and, as a very quiet person vho would normally blend into the background, I was also petrified. duly went back to bed, worried sick about my baby and trying not ɔ cry.

After fifteen minutes or so, a qualified nurse came to see me and ave me two sleeping tablets that were enormous – they looked like urple bombs!

"These will help you relax," I was told. They didn't. They made ne feel drugged, nauseous, and completely out of control with my reathing and the plans I had made to try and control my pain. The nly thing they *didn't* do was help me to sleep. I was in far too much ain to sleep and all I wanted to do was have some help or advice n what to do to feel more in control of the pain and keep my baby afe.

As soon as the morning staff took over, the staff nurse took one ɔok at me and said I needed to go straight up to the delivery suite. he then telephoned my husband to join me up there. Upon arrival, was shaved and given a full enema using a rubber tube and a large ɪg of water. I thought at this point that I was actually going to die. t was awful. The internal pressure was unbearable and at no point vas I given a choice about any of these procedures. Again, as such a quiet and reflective person, I did not challenge the professionals and thought this must have been the norm. When I was taken into the delivery room, I looked up and saw that the midwife who was about to deliver my baby was someone in the academic year below me at school. I was totally mortified! Could things get any worse?

I was the only person who was actually in the late stages of labour at that particular time, so there were (it seemed to me) a lot of students and trainee personnel coming in and out and talking to each other... But ignoring me and my husband. I can recall staff saying to each other how quiet I was and that I wasn't saying anything at all. I felt drugged, woozy, very sick, and unable to speak. I kept trying to "ride the pain" and sing songs in my head in order to focus. "This won't last forever," I told myself again and again and again!

After about two hours, I was given Pethidine via intramuscular injection into my thigh. As soon as this began to take effect, the nausea was at its peak. I tried to sit up, but it was too late, and I vomited a huge amount... It was everywhere! The midwife did her best to catch some with a small kidney dish that was only marginally successful! I lay back on the bed and I was sweating profusely by this stage. I could also feel uncontrollable pressure on my back and the sensation of everything "moving" inside me... Including the baby. My husband was given a wet flannel and told to wipe my forehead. The smell of the towelling fabric and the cold water that seeped through onto me was just the final straw that broke the (up until now) silent camel's back. I swore at my husband (and the world in general) with such vitriol and venom that it is still a standing family joke today, some decades later!

Twenty minutes later, after an episiotomy, my beautiful little dark-haired girl was born. Fast asleep. She was whipped from me and she was silent. I was shaking and thought that something terrible had happened to her. She had to have an injection to counteract the Pethidine that I was later told had crossed the placenta and affected her too. When she was deemed to be okay, she was passed to my husband. I just could not stop crying.

"You need to have your stitches," I was told. And that was that. I felt so cheated that after all that hard work, she was finally here, and I couldn't even control whether I was the first person to hold her. She was very jaundiced and yellow, spending ten days in hospital with me until she passed her blood test and we could go home. We were free at last... What an ordeal!

I later found out that I had been given what is known as a "sweep" at my original antenatal appointment without any knowledge of what it actually was. This was common practice (apparently) during the mid-'80s if the delivery wards were very quiet and being underutilised. I was so angry but later, when I had calmed down, I was just stunned. All that planning and preparation had been in vain. I was just another person giving birth and the choices I had wanted to make for the baby and for myself just didn't happen.

"Never again," I thought. "Never!"

I was so cross with myself for being so meek and compliant.

"When I have my second child, it will be so different," I vowed. And, two years later, it was. Thankfully.

Birth Journey D

My birth experience was completely the opposite to the one I had hoped for. While pregnant and attending my antenatal classes, the midwife told us about breathing techniques, demonstrated positions that would help with labour pains, and mentioned the birthing pool that the hospital offered. I was determined to do everything as naturally as possible and, since the pregnancy was low-risk, I qualified for the birthing pool. I envisioned myself bringing my son into the world while rippling waves lapped over my body, relatively pain-free thanks to a few yoga tricks, deep breathing, and gas and air… A euphoric hippy experience that I would be able to boast about for years to come!

Of course, my son wasn't playing ball and at 37 weeks he was still breech, despite my best efforts doing handstands and hanging backwards off the sofa. I was told that the hospital would like to try the ECV – External Cephalic Version – on the Thursday, a procedure where a trained doctor tries to turn the baby from the outside; I would be 37 weeks and 3 days pregnant. It carries a small risk that the baby might go into distress but, as my pregnancy had been healthy and uneventful, I decided to try it. Baby was already too big and while the doctor could lift his bum out of my pelvis, his head ended up somewhere near my ribs and he was impossible to manoeuvre (and it was all rather painful for me!) So I was sent home and told that the doctor would give me a date for a C-section the following Tuesday. I was a little disappointed.

I attended my next antenatal appointment and the doctor booked me in for a section on the Friday. I went to lunch with a friend and she'd bought a few bits and bobs for the baby. Husband came home, I started cooking dinner, I began to feel a niggling pain in my lower back… But put it down to all the walking I'd done that day. I asked Husband to rub my back for me – it didn't help. We ate and I went to bed with a hot water bottle. We usually watch TV in bed before we go to sleep, but my husband said he was too tired and was soon snoring peacefully. I was in agony and it suddenly dawned on me that the pain wasn't constant… It was a rhythmic pain. As baby was breech, I'd been told to call the hospital if my waters broke or if contractions started. So I gave them a ring and was told I'd better come in.

Upon examination, I was told my cervix was ripe and, not so long after that, I was in the second stage of labour. The pain of the contractions was surprisingly bearable, inconsistent with what I'd heard. After that, everything moved so fast. I was told to prepare to go to theatre and I don't remember feeling nervous, just excited and relieved that the big day was finally here!

Maybe it's because of the drugs they give you during the C-section, but my memory of the whole experience feels hazy. I remember my husband holding my hand and I remember the doctor peeking up over the curtain and saying, "Baby's bum is out!" I can remember holding my son for the first time, at 02:42, and the way he looked at me… I laughed with delight as he was placed close to me… I was in a love bubble. And I have to say, I didn't feel robbed of the birth experience because I hadn't had a "natural" labour (something I've heard a few other C-section mums complain of). The birth process was just the means to the end – finally meeting my son. No moment in my life so far could top that one (although his first smile and the sound of his first laugh came pretty close). I was smitten from the start.

My *recovery* from that emergency C-section was nothing short of brutal, however. Eight months later and I'm still not right! I didn't feel terrible pain in the hospital (the first time I sat up and walked around, the day after my section, I did vomit everywhere though). I went home after four days and tried to cope with being a mum… Determined to breastfeed, going out for walks, active from the get-go… Oh, trying to poo as well. With a C-section they move all your organs around and nothing works properly!

Two weeks into my recovery, I was struck with crippling pain. My scar was closed (no oozing or anything concerning there) but I could barely move. I went back to hospital and, because I had a fever, was kept in overnight and put on intravenous antibiotics. As I was breastfeeding, my son was kept in with me and they said they would weigh him, just to check he was okay. He hadn't gained back his birth weight and that issue became more important for me than the pain I was feeling. He had problems with his latch (possibly tongue tie) and I was panicking because I felt that I was failing as a mother. I had one job – feed the baby – and I couldn't do that! Aside from that, I was undergoing tests as my bloodwork showed an infection, but it wasn't in the incision that had closed. I had to go for an ultrasound, but they couldn't see anything wrong. I stayed in hospital for three days and it was a generally rotten experience.

Eventually, they let me out but in four weeks I was back again – referred by my doctor because of the same crippling pains. Again, my scar was completely closed and healed on the outside, so the infection was going on somewhere inside… But the scans were inconclusive, I had no waste product, my bowel was moving as it should, and everything seemed okay. This time I was visited by the surgeon, the lovely doctor who had seen me throughout my pregnancy, the physio department, and more… They still couldn't figure out why I had a recurrent infection. I was eventually allowed to go home.

Eight months down the line and despite having lost most of my baby weight (bar, let's say, 2kg), my stomach still has a huge bulge around my scar. Sometimes when I sit up or bend down too quickly it makes a farting or gurgling noise. It looks horrible and I can't wear anything tight. That's because I have an incisional hernia – a result of my C-section. I'm on the waiting list for a consultation and, eventually, an operation. I don't feel too confident about my body anymore, but I look at the bigger picture. My son is absolutely gorgeous. I'm totally besotted with him… Even when he's teething or done one of those massive stinky poos all up his back, even though I can't stay out late because he wants me there when he falls asleep, even though my whole life has changed and will never be the same again… This tiny boy looks at me with such love, his whole body gravitates towards me when he's sleeping next to me… He has such a need for me and me for him; I'd do it all again. I plan to have another, but I think this baby is always going to be my favourite, my first born, my mammy's boy.

Birth Journeys E & F

My first labour began in the textbook way… Although six days early, to my utter astonishment! (I was convinced she'd keep me waiting… As my husband will tell you, I'm not the most patient of people.) I'd been having Braxton-Hicks contractions for a few days and Husband had decided to work from home, just in case. We both lay on the bed, him on his laptop, tapping away, and me just trying to get some rest. And then... BOOM! I felt a strong force in my pelvis and my waters gushed. This was it. And I knew it! Husband came over to me, we looked at each other, and I cried. The realisation set in… This was the moment it was all about to change!

We drove to the hospital as my contractions had become more intense almost instantly. They were strong but infrequent by the time we got there. The midwife suggested we go and wait at home until they were more regular. We were at home for an hour before we decided to go back in. Now they were very strong and three minutes apart.

When we got back to hospital, they told me that I was 4cm dilated and sent me to the delivery suite. I remember having to stop once or twice for contractions in the corridors but, honestly, it's all a bit blurry. Time seemed to stand still. I had no concept of it.

I gave birth for the first time in Australia. Our delivery suite was really lovely – a big bed, bath, private shower, and toilet. It was a large room and all open-plan. There was atmospheric lighting. It felt nice.

The midwife was nice too, but not as warm as I'd hoped. The first midwife I'd seen was very motherly and I felt like I would've preferred to have her there. This one was pleasant enough though. I think her name was Kate but I can't remember. My mum and husband were both there through my whole labour. Mum was a massive support for me, but especially for my husband. It must be very hard for our partners to see us in so much pain.

Key moments that I can remember from my first labour include:

- Making sounds that I didn't know I could make or how I was even making them. I could hear the noise but I had no idea how I was doing it... I couldn't replicate it now!
- Feeling like I wanted to push so much but the midwife telling me not to just yet. This felt like the hardest part for me. Trying to get through a contraction without pushing felt like agony.
- Worrying my butt was about to explode. No joke.
- Asking for pain relief when I really didn't want any but feeling like I couldn't go on without some. I did have morphine, which is usual practice in Australia.
- Feeling relieved when I was told that I could push because the midwife could feel the head.
- Wanting to be naked the whole time!

Baby 1 came into the world after fourteen hours of labour, two hours of pushing, and an "almost" episiotomy (I was told they would give me one if I didn't get her out on that contraction. They anaesthetised but I got her out!) She was born at 05:04 on 27 February 2014 – my little girl. I felt like I'd had a wonderful experience! I was so happy that we got through it all unscathed (well,

I had a second-degree tear, but things could have been worse!) Everyone was healthy, we were both here, and now we could start our journey together. Little did I know that, with her, labour was the easy bit...!

*

This wonderful experience was trumped though. Second time around I decided, after a chat with a friend who's a midwife, to try for a home birth. I thought long and hard about the decision, discussed the idea with Husband (of course), and still had a look around the hospital, just in case. But I decided to go for it.

I was nervous. We hired a pool and I immediately felt like I had wasted the money that it cost because the likelihood of me actually going through with a home birth was slim. I mean, birth plans never go to plan... Do they?!

At 40 weeks and 5 days, I started having some stronger contractions after a day of Braxton Hicks-ing. My husband and I went to Aldi and bought an exercise ball as they had them in that week ("Ask Aldi and they shall deliver!" is our motto). I spent the evening bouncing on the ball, chatting away with Husband about whether or not I thought I was going to have a baby that night. At 22:00, I decided that I possibly was, so phoned the midwife. She said to call back in about an hour and to watch for my waters breaking. They didn't and after the phone call my contractions decided to stop!

When I called the midwife again, she advised to try and have a sleep but to wear a pad in case my waters broke... So I did just that! And managed to sleep until 03:00!

When I woke up, I was having a strong contraction again. I went to the toilet and thought that my waters might have broken but it wasn't as obvious as when I'd had my first baby – there wasn't a lot of water. I woke Husband. Another strong contraction. Called the midwife. Another strong contraction. She said she'd make her way over slowly as it would be a little while yet but to get the pool filling up.

By this time, it was about 04:00 and the contractions were coming thick and fast. Husband ran up and down the stairs, filling the pool and coming back to me for each contraction. He must have been exhausted! I was texting my best friend between contractions to let her know that this was it; I wanted her there. My parents were asleep in the next room. At 05:00, I started to panic that the midwife wouldn't get there in time. We called again but she arrived just after we'd called. Phew! She set up her little space in the living room, even though there wasn't much room left. She was really lovely and made me feel at ease. I felt very calm through most of the labour actually… Unlike in my first labour when I thought I was going to either die or explode! (All the drama.)

I found that being on all fours was most comfortable this time. During my first labour, I tried loads of positions but, this time, I seemed to know instinctively what I had to do. When the pool was finally full enough for me to get in at around 06:00, I got in – the relief was instant. Labouring felt so much easier. My best friend arrived at about 06:30. I had her on one hand and Husband on the other. We woke my mum at about 07:15 when I knew baby was coming… He was born at 07:27. Heaven. What an experience. We had done it! And at home.

Comparing my labours, I can now note a few differences:

- Second time round I felt much more in control. I could trust my body and that what I was feeling was normal, and I was therefore more relaxed. This had a lot to do with the fact that I'd done it once before!
- I had no drugs second time round and never felt the need for them. With my first labour I wanted *all* the drugs!
- My second labour was much quicker – fourteen hours vs four hours in terms of active labour.
- I didn't know the sex of my baby second time around and it was the best feeling to find out.

It took a few days to sink in that my birth plan had gone to plan. I don't take that for granted. I feel so lucky to have had that experience. So much so that I wonder, if I did have another baby, would I be brave enough to have them at home as well? It can't go to plan twice, surely? Can it…?!

Birth Journey G

As a man in a child-birthing situation you are commonly told that you are useless. You hear countless stories of men not knowing what to do and jokes about how it would've been better if they hadn't been there (not many funny jokes but I think they still count). My wife and I were determined for this not to be the case for us and so, before the birth of our first child, we prepared. We attended couple's prenatal yoga classes that focussed on things that both parties could do during labour to help with the pain, I learned all about the different stages of labour, downloaded a contraction timer app on two phones in case a battery died, we discussed the birth plan, she wrote the birth plan, I memorised the birth plan… I was ready. End-of-training-montage levels of ready.

When L day came, I can honestly say that I was useful. I knew what was going on and was able to be helpful and proactive throughout. There were some complications towards the end of the labour, and we did end up in theatre, but, once the baby was out and all were well, we viewed the labour as a generally positive experience in which we both played major roles.

When we started to prepare for the birth of our second child, I was quietly confident. We'd been through a labour with complications and it had been good. I brushed up on my massage skills and made sure my apps were still working… Now it was just a matter of time.

Labour started on our little one's due date. I timed the contractions as they built up, just like last time. As soon as they hit the "right" point, we called in childcare and, in the short forty minutes that it took for them to arrive, labour stopped. Completely. This happened on and off for twelve days. My wife barely slept as the contractions started every time she nodded off.

We tried everything we possibly could to get labour established – sweeps, spicy curries, bouncing on the birth ball, raspberry leaf tea, pineapple… Just a quick side-note to any midwives reading, "A session of gentle lovemaking… Even if you don't really feel like it," is not the advice to give to a woman who is 41 weeks pregnant, hasn't slept in ten days, throws up every day, and barely has enough energy to make it out of bed to go to the bathroom. Nothing says, "Horny!" quite like a full bladder, a bowl of sick next to the bed, and hallucinations caused by exhaustion.

After twelve days, we went through the same pattern of labour starting and then stopping until finally, we made it to the hospital with contractions in full force. They were at the same level as they'd been when my wife was about 5cm dilated during her first labour and I was excited – as far as I was concerned, this was happening now. We got into triage where the midwife checked and reported that she was only 2cm dilated. A bit of back and forth later and we were sent to walk around the hospital, at 06:00. I have never seen my wife look as hurt as she did right then. I could see the resignation in her eyes. I know how strong my wife is – her strength of will and strength of character put me to shame – and this was the closest I'd ever seen her to defeat. I tried everything I could – the massages that helped with the pain so well last time hurt her this time, my knowledge of how a labour progresses didn't help when the labour wasn't progressing normally, and my contraction timer was jumping around like no-one's business. I tried everything I could to tell her that she could do this, but I had nothing to offer except encouragement.

What happened next was a blur... We settled on a sofa with a drink in a coffee shop and spent ten minutes planning when we were going to go home. My wife dozed off for five minutes and then woke up in the middle of actively pushing. We were rushed into a room with two midwives, no records, no time for gas and air, and, within two minutes of getting into that room, the baby arrived. My wife deteriorated rapidly and, at the time, all I knew was that there were far too many doctors in the room, far too much blood, and that my wife was in pain.

I had the baby now. I was pushed up against the corner of the room as the doctors and nurses did what NHS staff do so well. There were about fifteen people all acting together and I could just about understand what was happening, but I couldn't get close to my wife, I couldn't help, or explain, or do anything! A few minutes later, my wife was taken to theatre and we made damn sure we told each other we loved each other as she was wheeled away. The room that had been a frenzy of activity just a few moments before, with my wife in the middle, suffering, was now empty.

I didn't move from my corner for some time. I had too many emotions to deal with at once. I was terrified of what was happening to my wife. I didn't know why they were taking her to theatre but, given the blood loss, I could easily imagine the worst. At the same time, I had our son in my arms, a small child who, at that point, only had me. I couldn't, and still can't to this day, reconcile the combination of feeling so scared, so helpless, and so useless, but, at the same time, feeling love for my newborn child and understanding just how dependent he was on me.

I should add at this point that all ended well. My wife came around from her general anaesthetic a few hours later. She had lost a lot of blood, about two and a half litres, very quickly, and they needed to take her to theatre to stop the bleeding and give her a few blood transfusions. Once she came around, she was greeted by a little baby plopped onto her and, after those eventful first few hours, we experienced our first proper moment together as a family.

Birth Journey H

I've since described labour as running marathons but not knowing how many you have to run. In a row. You finish one, only to find out there's another… And no-one can tell you how many there are 'til you reach the finish.

Yet now I'm just remembering making this comparison, not the event itself. Would I remember it was that hard? It seems like another life, so hopefully I can be honest…

I'd felt pretty prepared, armed with antenatal classes and hypnobirthing techniques BOOM but once the contractions got intense BOOM I was BOOM catapulted into another world where BOOM I had no time or mental space to access calmly my box of BOOM tricks BOOM I can't do this BOOM I'm never ever doing this again BOOM why BOOM did we put ourselves in this scenario, no-one made us choose this moment… Were just some of the negative thoughts I had during labour. After all that positive preparation! The pain was beyond what I expected, far beyond.

Funny I wasn't scared of the pain; I just couldn't bear not being able to escape it. I never once thought to ask for an epidural, I just thought I might be stuck in the room for eternity, that my baby might never come out.

I'm so grateful to the midwife for believing in my strength. She pushed me (kindly) to keep going, she knew what my body was capable of more than I did.

I think it was good not to fear the birth but a massive shock to find it unbelievably painful and exhausting. I repeat – I did not think I could keep going!

It was very light in the week leading up – during the day I was impatient and wanted labour to start and, at night, in the dark, I was scared. Maybe my body knew to wait.

I truly thought it was a disaster during the labour. I felt like I'd failed, like I didn't know what to do, or that I might not get my baby out. Even after (for a day or so), I thought it was a failure. Then I saw, in my notes, boxes ticked for "non-caesarean", "no intervention". Not that they would have signified failure but, at that point, I realised – I did it! I got a baby out of my body. Using movement, breath, noise, physical support from my husband and midwife, a bit of water (well, a lot – a pool full – but not for long) – I got her out.

Her! Yes, a real person came out. I did not feel emotional, or tender. It was a physical/body response to a physical/body process of delivering her into the world outside my body. I'd had that through the whole pregnancy. I felt so connected and aware of my body – no tears of emotion at the first scan! Just a sense of normality.

So. I grew to enjoy the birth retrospectively. To love it again and be grateful for such a *huge unique* thing to undergo. Yes, I pooed. No, I didn't care. Yes, I was completely naked. No, I didn't care.

It was a "normal" labour. Quite long. Not hugely. Very painful – but apparently not impossible. No intervention.

But in reality – I had a baby who had been so low for weeks that everything was already sore and a pelvic floor that was used to squeezing, not relaxing.

Little things came back to me… How delicious a sip of water was, how sweaty I was, how the midwife whispering made me think something bad was happening…

Yes, I would do it again. Despite being 100% sure I never would ever want to…

What a crazy thing. What amazing bodies.

It was horrendous… And amazing.

Birth Journeys I & J

In preparation for birth my husband and I attended NCT classes. The girls in the group, as our maternity leaves started and we anxiously awaited our new arrivals, had got into the habit of meeting up on Friday afternoons for tea and cake. The due date for our first baby was 14 June 2015. By Friday 26 June, there was still no sign of arrival, in spite of a sweep the day before, and an induction was booked in for Sunday 28. During this weekly NCT gathering, a few of the Dads joined us and we moved on to the pub. My husband and I were joking that perhaps we ought to go on a ride on our tandem the next day to try and hurry things along!

In the early hours of Saturday morning, it became clear that a tandem ride probably wasn't going to be necessary. The contractions started at around 03:00. We were nervous and excited and pretty impatient for things to get going, setting up the TENS machine and the "Contraction Timer" app. I kept active, bouncing around on my birthing ball, and we managed to go for a little wander around mid-morning (I haven't been able to walk along that path since without remembering!) I didn't have much of an appetite but tried to pick at things to keep my energy up.

I first phoned the hospital at around 16:00. By now, the contractions were coming steadily and although not entirely regular, I think they were usually around every six minutes. I was a bit concerned about the journey to hospital. We live in a fairly rural location about half an hour from Derby, but I'd actually chosen to give birth at the Queen's Medical Centre (QMC) in Nottingham – I see a hepatology consultant there as I have a (not particularly serious) liver condition. He'd wanted me to be at the QMC in case there were complications relating to my condition but, in fact, I'd been absolutely fine. What this did mean was that it was going to take us nearly an hour to get to hospital.

When I spoke to the midwife, however, she didn't seem at all concerned about the length of the journey. "You're a first-time mum," I was told. "You've got a while to go yet. Turn your TENS machine off and have a bath." Trying not to feel too despondent, I followed this advice – although without the TENS machine the pain felt much worse. After my bath, I put it back on but tried not to turn it up too much as I probably had a lot longer to go.

My recollections of the rest of the evening are a bit blurry. The contractions got stronger and more painful but still weren't particularly regular – sometimes closer together, sometimes further apart. Then I was sick. I phoned the hospital again at around 23:00. The contractions hadn't really grown much closer together, but they were feeling more intense. My waters hadn't broken and the midwife I spoke to still didn't think I needed to come in. She asked, "Are you not coping with the pain?" Rightly or wrongly, I interpreted this to mean that she thought I should be able to cope, so I said I could probably manage to wait a bit longer.

By around 03:00, having been awake for twenty-four hours, we were both stressed and exhausted. My husband started worrying about being able to drive safely to hospital having had no sleep and he went to have a bit of a rest, so he'd be ready to drive us when needed. He did this with my agreement but it was a mistake – without his supportive presence, panic started to set in and the pain became overwhelming. The contractions still weren't any closer together, but I phoned the hospital and told them I was coming in as I was worried that I couldn't feel the baby moving. I don't think this was really true; I'd just got to the point where I didn't want to stay at home any longer.

I was dreading the journey, but the contractions actually seemed to be waning a bit and I only had a couple in the car. At that time in the morning, the A52 was unsurprisingly deserted and it only took us about forty minutes to arrive.

We parked right at the front of the hospital and I walked in. The midwife took one look at me and kindly said that she didn't think I was in active labour, but they'd have a look and give me a sweep to see if they could hurry things along before we went home.

After a short wait, she examined me and her attitude changed.

"You're going to love me in a minute," she said. "I think you're about 7cm dilated. You're not going anywhere. You're going to have a baby today!"

I felt enormous relief and was also quite proud of myself – I'd managed all that time on my own. I asked about using a birthing pool, one was available, and so we were shown through to a pool room in the birthing centre and introduced to the midwife who'd be looking after us. (I'm embarrassed and surprised that I can't remember her name as she was lovely!) We were excited, taking photos and setting up music. I got into the pool and sat back, feeling pretty lucky that things were all going so well…

One thing was missing though – the contractions seemed to have stopped. I only had one in the pool and that didn't really mount up in the way that they'd begun to at home. Our midwife initially didn't seem that worried and encouraged me to keep moving around in the pool. She also tried using essential oils to kick-start things again. However, when I'd had no further contractions for about an hour, the decision was taken that they were going to examine me again and that they'd have to break my waters to try and re-start things. I was a bit upset that things had stalled but, of course, was happy to do whatever was needed.

When she examined me, this midwife said she thought I was probably only 6cm dilated, rather than the 7cm estimated during my first examination. Then when she broke my waters, there was meconium in them, which meant an immediate transfer to the maternity ward. (My care had been consultant-led throughout my pregnancy because of my liver condition but, as there hadn't been any problems, the initial plan was to give birth in the midwife-led birthing centre.)

I was told to lie on a bed and was hooked up to a monitor. The doctors came in and discussed the situation. As they were concerned that the baby was in distress, they wanted to put me on the Syntocinon drip to kick-start labour. I can't remember exactly what timings they said but it was something like I needed to do another four hours of contractions with the contractions coming every four minutes. Whatever the figures were, at that moment, it just seemed impossible. I was exhausted and panicking and just had no faith whatsoever in my ability to carry on, particularly as it seemed I had to stay lying on the bed and not move round as before.

My birth plan had always been to have as natural a labour as possible, using a birthing pool, but our NCT course had left me well-informed about the other options available. In particular, one of the dads on the course just happened to be a consultant anaesthetist and he'd spoken quite a lot in the session on pain relief. His advice was that if you arrive at the stage where you need the drip and think you might want an epidural, then it's best to have it as early as possible – once you're in the throes of the extremely strong contractions brought on by the drip, then it becomes very difficult for the anaesthetist to administer the epidural. So, in the days leading up to the date set for my induction, I'd decided that if I needed the drip, I'd probably ask for an epidural. And now, feeling exhausted and disheartened, it seemed like the most sensible option. Weirdly, the anaesthetist who gave me my epidural said that our NCT dad had taught him how to do it!

I must admit that there will probably always be a small part of me that wishes I hadn't had to resort to the epidural and that I'd been able to carry on without it. But, deep down, I know that, at the time, it was the right decision. It gave me a chance to rest – I even dozed for a couple of hours before they told me it was time to push – and I've no doubt that I might not have coped with the next stage as well as I did without the break that the pain relief had given me.

We were very lucky that our designated midwife stayed with us the entire time (I think she was actually fairly junior so perhaps hadn't been given a particularly heavy caseload). She monitored my contractions (as I could no longer feel them!) and the baby's heartbeat throughout, and she was a very reassuring presence.

After about four hours, the doctors returned and agreed with our midwife that it was now time to start pushing. This felt very strange – because of the epidural I still couldn't feel anything at all, so there wasn't the usual build up or desire to push. The midwife had to watch the monitor for the contractions and tell me when to push, which seemed very odd! The doctors informed me that because I'd had the epidural, it was likely that I'd need further intervention. I'm sure that they were just trying to prepare me but, in my emotional state, this almost sounded like a threat. I was pretty determined that I was *not* going to need forceps or anything else… And I really went for it! It was very strange not feeling any sensation at all, but I pushed as hard as I could.

There was a growing sense of tension – the team were concerned that they couldn't always get a reading on the baby's heartbeat and so were calling for the paediatricians to be on standby. In contrast to this worry was the hilarious sound of my husband joining in with the noises I was making while pushing (I think he just felt he had to do something!) It was an odd situation. Not feeling anything made this stage seem almost a bit anticlimactic – I was pushing when instructed rather than following the more natural cues we'd expected.

But, to everybody's surprise, in spite of all the warnings about extra help, after only thirty minutes of pushing, our baby was suddenly there. As he appeared on the bed, I remember the senior midwife proclaiming, "There's nothing wrong with that baby!" All concerns seemed to evaporate. For some reason, I'd been certain through pregnancy that we were having a boy and when somebody asked what I'd had, I didn't actually look… I just knew he was a "he". Our Baby. He was born at 18:00 on the Sunday night – 39 hours after I'd first felt a contraction.

I'd like to be able to write something about the delivery of the placenta but, to be honest, I can't really remember anything about it! I do remember them telling me that I didn't need a further "anti-D" injection as Baby had also tested as rhesus negative. But mainly, I remember us just sitting in the room holding our baby. Our lovely midwife had reached the end of her shift, so we had a bit of a wait before the new one came in to stitch me up (I had a second-degree tear, although, thanks to epidural, wasn't in any discomfort).

So there we have it. My first labour was very long and, at times, very stressful. But, in many ways, I was lucky – I was able to make a well-informed decision about pain relief, it worked, and then I had a very quick second stage that delivered a healthy baby. Unfortunately, for a long time afterwards, I think my memories of this were tempered by breastfeeding complications. This is another story for another time but what I will say is that our feeding complications were the start of a downward spiral that took me a long time to get out of. So when I became pregnant again, I knew that things needed to be different. And that a more positive birth experience would be a good start.

The first thing I did was ask to give birth at Derby, our nearest hospital, rather than having to worry about travelling further to Nottingham. As there hadn't been any complications with my liver the first time round, my hepatology consultant was happy with this decision (but he did refer me to the Derby hepatology team, just in case).

On a friend's recommendation, I signed up for a couple of terms of Daisy Active Birthing Classes – they're a mixture of antenatal education, yoga, and hypnobirthing. There's a lot of focus on maintaining a positive mindset and on the importance of mothers being able to make their own choices during labour and beyond.

I must admit, I was a bit sceptical about all the positive affirmations, or at least sceptical that they would work for me – I'm pretty good at hanging on to the negative sometimes. However, the course leader was incredibly supportive and I was able to discuss my fears about breastfeeding and about not being listened to. Her advice enabled me to accept what had happened in my first labour and afterwards, and to begin to see the positive in my previous choices, instead of just beating myself up. She also gave me the confidence to seek advice and help with breastfeeding in advance and practical plans were put in place.

I don't know how much can be attributed to a more positive mindset but, if you'd asked me before my second labour how I'd wanted things to go, then this birth would have been pretty much it.

Our first piece of luck was timing. Given that our first baby was two weeks late, I was fairly confident that our second baby, who was due 31 August 2018, would be too. I had an appointment with my hepatology consultant in Nottingham on 28 August, so I asked my mum (who lives four hours away) to come up and babysit while I went to the QMC. That evening, my husband, Mum, and I sat watching *The Great British Bake Off*, laughing at the fact that the baby appeared to be performing an acrobatic routine inside me. But perhaps the baby was just gearing up… At about 04:00, I awoke to a twinge that I very quickly realised was the start of my second labour.

This time round I didn't jump straight into action but tried to stay in bed and rest a bit. Lying and sitting down soon became too uncomfortable though, and I got up and started moving round the room. My husband was very surprised when he realised what was happening. He went and got my birthing ball so we could stay in our room, rather than disturbing the others, and he helped me set up the TENS machine. He also got me some breakfast… I thought I wanted it but then, about an hour later, I was sick.

When we'd talked about my first labour and how we wanted things to be different second time round, one of the key things for my husband was getting to hospital earlier. He repeatedly said, "We should have gone in after you were sick." So when I was sick this time, he saw it as a sign that we really should get going. My contractions were now coming about every four or five minutes and I couldn't really talk through them. We tried to call the hospital but couldn't get through. My husband just said, "We'll call them on the way." He was adamant. So after a cuddle and a bit of an explanation for our first baby, we left him with Grandma and off we went.

Our second piece of luck was that even though we left the house at 08:30 on a weekday, there seemed to be very little traffic on the roads. I called the hospital again from the car and was just told to make our way to the labour ward. I had a few contractions in the car – they definitely weren't slowing down this time – but I was able to breathe through them reasonably easily.

Upon our arrival at the hospital there was absolutely no questioning about whether or not I needed to be there. We were shown straight into a room and introduced to our midwife (whose name I can't remember either, sorry!) She didn't examine me straight away but left us to settle in.

I think when she did examine me, I was about 5cm dilated but it didn't really seem to matter – I felt like they were taking me much more seriously this time, it was less like I had to prove myself. She suggested that I might like some pain relief and saw to getting me some gas and air. The one sticking point was that my care was consultant-led and I'd been on medication throughout pregnancy (my usual medication – ursodeoxycholic acid – that I take every day). The midwife wanted me to be monitored continuously. I wanted to be able to move around and keep standing (not least because sitting and lying down were pretty painful by this point!) So we compromised – I was on the monitor but standing by the edge of the bed. This was the difference – second time round I was more aware of the choices I could make and was more confident in expressing my wishes. Consequently, I felt much more in control throughout.

The contractions progressed steadily over the next few hours and, while she was always there in the background, our midwife gave me space to get on with it. My memories are a bit hazy. I do remember the midwife being concerned about me eating something, so my husband fed me Jelly Babies, bits of Kit Kat, and toast. At one point, the doctors came, and I remember standing there between contractions telling them that I was pretty pleased with how things were going. They said it wasn't going to take as long as last time and probably would all be over in around six hours. We did ask about using a birthing pool but there wasn't one available. To be honest, I got the distinct impression that the midwife wouldn't have been keen even if there had been a pool – things were progressing well and I don't think she wanted any disturbances or distractions. I felt I was managing well, so that was fine with me too. I remember when our midwife went on a break that another colleague brought me a wheat heat pack that was helpful for my back.

Several things I'd learned during the antenatal classes helped me through the next few hours. Simple things like not biting down on the gas-and-air mouthpiece because tightening your jaw also tightens your pelvic floor. There had been much emphasis on treating each contraction as a wave and, for some reason, this was something that I was really able to work with. As each contraction came, I took a big breath of gas and air and then clicked the "BOOST" button on the TENS machine – when turned up to the max, this felt like someone was pushing me and supporting my back. I imagined that I was getting up on a surfboard and riding over the top of each "wave"! I've always been completely rubbish at surfing, so that was definitely the gas and air talking, but somehow this visualisation enabled me to zone out completely of what was going on around me.

I was determined to stand throughout, but my feet did start to ache and I was helped to kneel on the bed – I was still upright but could take the pressure off my feet for a bit. Though things were progressing well, by 14:00 my waters still hadn't broken, and I don't think the baby's head was quite as far down as it should have been for the next stage. Our midwife suggested that she should break them as that would probably hurry things along a bit. She was right – once this was done, things progressed very quickly indeed. The contractions became really intense and, for a minute, I lost my focus, panicked a little, and took in a bit too much gas and air. She took the mouthpiece off me for a second and told me to calm down. Then, something in my head just clicked – I knew I had to switch to the next type of breathing I'd been taught in the Daisy classes (inhaling and then exhaling like you're blowing a candle out) and then carried on as before.

I remember the midwife saying, "Tell me when you feel like you need to push." And then suddenly, I did need to push.

I was standing up and she told me to move back to kneeling on the bed so that they could catch the baby more easily. I do remember thinking, "You want me to move now?! You must be joking!" But they all helped me and I managed it, and suddenly the head was out, and then the baby was there, and my husband was telling me we had another boy. He was born at 15:02. I think I only had to push for ten minutes. I'll probably never feel as strong or as proud of myself as I did when I sat there holding him. We hadn't fully decided on a name – there were two in the running – but when I looked at him, I knew which one was right.

The next bit didn't quite go according to plan. As everything had gone so smoothly so far, the midwife was very keen that I should have a natural third stage and deliver the placenta without the aid of the Syntocinon injection. However, it just didn't want to come away. I tried moving around and, at her suggestion, sitting on the toilet but nothing seemed to work. I was feeling pretty exhausted and as the euphoria of the birth wore off, I remember feeling like I really didn't want to deal with any more pain... And this hurt a lot! Afterwards, my husband said that this was the only point in the whole of the proceedings when he was really worried about me – I'd gone as white as a sheet and started looking pretty unwell. In the end, I asked if I could have the injection. The placenta did come away after that, though they recorded that the membranes were a bit ragged. I did lose quite a lot of blood, so I was kept in overnight and sent home with iron tablets... But none of that mattered. My husband, our baby, and I spent a very relaxed afternoon together in the room on the labour ward. Baby had his various checks and then, quite late in the evening, I was taken upstairs. The ward was peaceful. As the feeding specialists had written up the feeding plan we'd devised, there were no worries about Baby getting enough milk. I remember lying with our baby in my arms early the next morning, not quite believing how easy everything had been. I feel very privileged that I got to find out what a wonderfully empowering experience giving birth can be.

Birth Journey K

I wish my story was one of a beautiful water birth or one where I starred as a one-push wonder… Instead, my labour ended up filled with feelings of fear, frustration, and forceps!

My due date came and went, and I was booked in for an induction twelve days past my due date. "This is great!" I thought. "I know when my baby is going to be born!" And my husband and I promptly started looking up famous people born on that date… I was so excited!

Sure enough, I was given an ambulatory induction method, Propress, and was allowed to go home until things started moving. Within a few hours, my cervix was on fire and bleeding, and the induction thing fell out during a trip to the loo! I went back into hospital that night hoping that they would make everything okay and administer the next step. They said I'd had a rare reaction to the product, which had caused the pain, but that the hormone within it had actually worked as I was now 3cm dilated. They said they wanted me to go home and wait for labour to progress naturally; the next step would be to have my waters broken…

Now I want to preface the rest of my story by saying that I think the NHS is a brilliant thing. We are so lucky in this country to have access to free medical care and I have huge respect for anyone who works in the service… Can you feel a "but" coming? Unfortunately, thanks to a handful of midwives, an experience that should have been magical and centred around my wants and needs, ended up being truly traumatic, and I've never felt more invisible in my life. It took staff twenty-seven hours to find me a bed in the delivery suite so that I could have my waters broken. I know that sentence is a simple one and, at a glance, seems to contain just a number… But I want you to picture me sitting, mostly alone, on a hospital bed for *twenty-seven hours*, watching the door to the ward, just waiting for a midwife to walk in and tell me that it was time to meet my baby. Every time she walked in my heart raced, but she instead went to another patient or just came to do my obs. I'd exhausted all possible activities that one can do on a ward. My husband and I had even learnt the little guide explaining the different uniforms that staff wear and had tested each other when we spotted one. It was impossible to sleep in that room; there were four bays and women were coming in and out in various stages of labour. I felt like Rachel in *Friends* when women who'd come in after her were pushing before she was! This must have happened to me about eight times since I was first admitted. I'd sent my husband home to sleep so at least one of us was well-rested. I tried to be all independent and not mind being the only person alone on the ward but, in reality, I've never felt lonelier in my life… I pulled my curtains shut and just cried and cried. Add to this the pressure of being messaged every five minutes by friends and family asking if Baby had arrived yet, and the fact that my mum had already been off work for two weeks as she'd pre-booked it off expecting the baby to be here on his due date… She was due back at work in a few days and still no grandson for her. I felt awful. I felt like a failure.

Fourteen days past my due date at 19:00 was finally my turn! The midwife came in and said a bed was available. As I was having my waters broken, I needed one-to-one midwife care and they'd not had the staffing to allow this until now. I was introduced to my midwife and shown around my delivery room. It felt amazing knowing that this was the room where I'd meet my baby and a relief knowing that I wouldn't be leaving that room again without him! My husband got straight on the TV and whacked on *Hairy Bikers*. There are some things you never expect when you're expecting… In my case, watching Si and Dave whilst contracting! Wait, I'm getting ahead of myself…

So, by this point, I hadn't slept for more than a few hours across a sixty-hour period and was already exhausted, but I was also so excited that it was all finally happening. My adrenaline levels were sky high and I was so pumped for this! A nice nurse came in and broke my waters (after missing the first time with the little hook and accidentally cutting my clitoris… I digress). A waterfall of amniotic fluid drenched the bed below me. I'd been worrying in late pregnancy that I might not notice my waters breaking and might just mistake it for wetting myself a bit… I can safely say that there's no mistaking that sensation! But therein lies the rub – because I'd been induced in this way, I had to be strapped up to a monitor for the rest of my labour. They were tracking my contractions and also Baby's heartbeat. I was limited to lying on a bed, which was not part of my birth plan and was something I was pretty upset about. I'd envisioned walking around, leaning over the bed, and bouncing on gym balls. I'd also read that giving birth lying down increased the risk of tearing and was a very unnatural position to push in. I'd wanted to squat, stand, or kneel on the bed. Alas, something else that was not to go as planned.

My labour then progressed very quickly. I was soon having regular, painful contractions and by 23:00, I was already 7cm dilated (from being just 3cm at the point of my waters breaking at 19:00). During pregnancy I'd decided I didn't want any major pain relief as

I wanted to remain completely compos mentis, so up till now I'd just been using breathing techniques and quite a lot of swear words. But the pain was getting intense, so I buckled and went on gas and air. It made me feel really light-headed, so I tried to use it only when I really needed to at first. By the end, I was chewing on the pipe pretty much constantly, but we'll get to that later...

Around 01:00, I started feeling an urge to push. I'd read about the foetal ejection reflex and this felt like that. My midwife, however, insisted it wasn't time and that I wasn't dilated enough (even though I'd not been examined in at least an hour). With me being a first-time mum and her a skilled practitioner, I assumed she was right and suppressed the urge. I asked her to examine me again shortly afterwards and, lo and behold, I was 10cm. But by then, the urge to push had lessened – I'd missed that magical window that nature had opened up for me. I started pushing with my contractions like she was telling me to do and it was all systems go. After an hour or so, my husband and midwife gasped and said they could see the head and that my baby had lots of dark hair. I felt euphoric and thought I was minutes away from meeting my little fella! But, no matter how hard I pushed, it just wasn't happening – he wasn't coming out. I'd been pushing for two hours now and was starting to get extremely upset and exhausted. This is when things started to get a bit scary.

Another midwife was called in to examine me and give a second opinion. She was a bit of a battle-axe and certainly didn't mince her words. This is the moment that sticks out for me in my labour, the moment that still fills me with angry tears when I remember it… She said, "Well, it's quite simple – you're not pushing." Yes, that's right, after two hours of excruciating pushing and the baby *apparently* nearly crowning, I *apparently* was just not trying hard enough. This was a bitter pill to swallow. Even my husband, who is normally of a quiet, shy disposition, and who, in a typical British way, would never question a trained professional to their face, actually asked her if she was joking. My midwife who had been with me the whole time stayed quiet and didn't stand up for me either, despite having watched said two hours of pushing. I assume there was something political going on there.

Anyway, she told me to push more "through my bum". This to the woman who had piles the size of Jupiter! I did as I was told and carried on trying. Still nothing. I was now screaming with pain; the second midwife told me to be quiet and said that I was being dramatic. At this point, I actually asked her not to speak to me like that and requested that she left. Even in my Entonox-induced state I could tell that this woman was being downright out of order. I mean, come on, things not to say to a woman in labour! "You're not pushing!", "Be quiet!"… I don't think so.

I was so distressed, and no-one was listening to me. I was made to feel like a stupid little girl who didn't know what she was doing. Anyone who knows me knows that I do my research and study up over anything… But can anyone really ever be 100% prepared for their first labour?

They examined the baby internally and said that he was slightly turned, which could explain why it was so difficult to push him out. They would try a ventouse. I'd need an episiotomy and they'd need to call the surgeon in, which could take a while. Not even Si and Dave's cheeky faces could cheer me up now.

The room filled up very quickly with midwives, the surgeon, and nurses. The surgeon was clearly stressed and talking about an emergency that she'd been called away from for this. Again, another thing not to say to a woman in labour – that she's keeping you from something. Was I not an emergency? My legs were unceremoniously shoved into stirrups, an episiotomy carried out, and the ventouse inserted. They told me that I still had to push (seriously?! What is even the point of a vacuum if you still have to push?!), so we waited for the next contraction. Baby still wasn't coming out. Next contraction… Still nothing. Same for the one after. They removed the ventouse and declared it time to move on to forceps. By now, I felt like I was about to break, both physically and mentally. I'd been through three days of failed inductions and interventions. My husband looked terrified; I caught a glance of him standing in the corner, looking like he was witnessing something horrific. He later described the experience as "watching a triage room at the Battle of the Somme". This is also when I started chewing on that gas-and-air pipe and The Battle Axe actually took it from me and said she thought I'd had enough. Simply. Not. Okay. They told me to push again with the next contraction to help the forceps work and, sure enough, the moment came, and I pushed so hard I thought I was going to prolapse… But then, finally, my baby was born.

This tiny, bloody, amazing thing was placed on my chest and my husband and I both burst into tears. I was feeling a thousand emotions at once – relief that he was finally here and that he was okay, overwhelmed by the fact he was the most beautiful thing I'd ever seen in my life, and truly and utterly exhausted. I held him while my placenta was delivered but then Baby had to be taken away while I had my stitches done (I was in too much pain and needed to go back on the gas and air). So, for the next forty-five minutes, I had to watch my husband walk around the room with our newborn son while I was being seen to… I just wanted to hold him and do skin-to-skin and try to get him latched on… But, yet again, I felt useless.

When it was finally all over (and I'd had a shower, a good cuddle, a cup of tea, and a good cry), when it was just me, my husband, and our baby, it hit me that I was really a mother now. I felt wonderful and, as most mothers will tell you, that feeling of devotion makes all the pain worth it. Mine was not an easy ride and, truthfully, I'm still not recovered physically ten weeks later, but I have Baby and he is my world now…

I didn't think love like this was possible.

Birth Journey L

Friend 1: I did loads of prep for labour. Like, I did hypnobirthing and stuff… I went to baby yoga and the teacher was very much talking about breathing exercises and, "You can dance through labour if you want," and I thought, "This is exactly what I'm going to do! I'm going to be a Birth Earth Mother!" And then, with my first, it worked really *really* well… I was all over that birth ball and breathing like some sort of tantric pro! Husband came to some classes with me, so he knew exactly what to do – reminding me to breathe, gently pressing my hips, looking into my eyes… And I felt like we were one. It's so bloody cheesy but the whole "bring the baby into the world with the loving vibes in which they were conceived" idea was very much on the cards for us. But then, with my second, I felt like my pelvis was being prized opened by a nutcracker. No amount of dancing was going to get rid of that pain. And I didn't want anyone, *anyone* to touch me.

Friend 2: I had antenatal yoga, which I really liked and, yes, the instructor taught us some nice breathing-type exercises. In my head, before labour started, my plan was just to breathe through it as much as I could and have a bit of gas and air. I wanted to have a water birth, or at least be in the pool for the first bit.

Friend 1: I really *really* wanted a water birth.

Friend 2: I'd never… really… experienced *pain* properly before. I've never broken a leg, you know, or had a horrible accident or anything like that, so I wasn't sure how it was going to go. My waters broke at about 22:00 on the Monday and they were brown. And I was like, "Oh. That's not supposed to happen." So I rang the midwife unit and said, "Hello! My waters have broken and they're a bit brown and do you need to have a look?" And they said, "Yes, yes, come in." At that point, I sort of assumed they were going to check it out and say, "Nothing's happening, come back in five hours," or whatever. I didn't think I'd be in for the night because my sister was staying with us. So I was like, "Ooh! We're going to hospital now! Probably see you later this evening!" But they had a look and said, "Yes, there's definitely some meconium in the amniotic fluid, so you need to stay in, and we might have to induce to get things going." But then… So hang on… Yes, I arrived at the midwife-led unit where I had intended to give birth. But because of *that* they sent me up to the consultant-led unit, just at the other end of the same hospital. So I still wasn't sure whether it was happening now or not?! I kept thinking, "Oh, they're just going to monitor me for a bit and then send me home," because I hadn't had any contractions yet. So I was in a room in the consultant-led unit. And then they said, "We need to get things going because of the meconium in the amniotic fluid," and then just sort of wandered off for like an hour?! And I was like, "Am I going to be prepped for a C-section?!" and "How urgent is this?!"

Friend 1: At that point I'd have expected some sort of rapid-fire induction prep…

Friend 2: Yeah! They got as far as getting me to sign the consent to have… whichever drug it is that starts the labour. But by then, I'd actually

72

started having contractions myself. So they didn't do that in the end. I said to the midwife, "I'm having sort of pangs and I think my contractions have started." And she was like, "Ooh, they're not contractions." And I'm like, "WELL, SOMETHING'S HAPPENING IN INTERVALS AROUND MY ABDOMEN!" I didn't know if they were *contractions* because I could still talk. But they must have been contractions because what else would I have been having? So she wasn't very impressed. I never got round to mentioning, "Can I have a water birth?" because I wasn't sure if it was happening now or not. And I kind of just sort of forgot and I didn't know if there was a birth pool in the consultant-led bit.

One of the things I *was* worried about... Well, I didn't say that I *didn't* want to be in a consultant-led unit, but I did want to avoid as many interventions as possible. But, in the end, actually, you can have a gentle midwife-led birth at the consultant-led unit. Literally, some doctors popped in for five minutes, just to do their rounds or whatever, just to say, "Hello!", and then left again. And that was the only time I saw a doctor. Erm, I think... No, maybe actually one did turn up... Hmm, I don't know, see, I had other things to concentrate on! I think a doctor did turn up at one point. But again, I don't think she actually *did* anything. I think it was all the midwives who were actually looking after me. I've suddenly got this memory of a woman in scrubs being there and I can't remember if she administered something...

Friend 1: I honestly couldn't remember a single person...

Friend 2: This was what I was worried about! That I wouldn't be able to remember enough detail to be able to say anything...

Friend 1: We saw some friends recently... He's an anaesthetist and he was on call around the time I was due to give birth and he was like, "If you need an epidural, it might be me!" Could you imagine?! Anyway, he was asking about the team that had come in to debrief after I'd had my haemorrhage, and he asked, "Was there a lady with blonde hair? Was there a lady with glasses?" And I replied, "I. Have. No. Idea." The world and his wife could've walked through with trumpets.

Friend 2: Yeah, I didn't know what was happening... In the end, I did have some drugs... What did I have drugs for? I had gas and air for a while, which I don't think I did properly. But I didn't like the "floating away" feeling, I didn't like feeling like I wasn't there, so I probably didn't use it properly... But I think it did help.

Friend 1: I bloody loved gas and air. It was so *so* good and provided so much relief. When pregnant with my second, I fantasised about it and as soon as I arrived on that delivery suite, I shouted, "WHERE'S THE GAS AND AIR? I NEED IT NOW!"

Friend 2: The midwife suggested I have some Pethidine and I thought, "Yeah, that actually sounds like a really good idea." I had to have two doses of that in the end.

Friend 1: Did it work?

Friend 2: Yeah, I think so... I did puke. That was one of the reasons why I didn't want Pethidine was because I didn't want to vomit because I hate *hate* vomiting. But I threw up anyway, so I thought, "Might as well have some Pethidine now!" Yeah, I threw up several times. That was horrible.

Friend 1: What was your best bit of labour? Was there any part that you were really proud of?

Friend 2: Well, the baby came out! Hmm…

The contractions started and then they got worse and that took hours, all night basically. The contractions started by midnight probably and she wasn't born till 13:30, so it was *all* night contracting. I was mostly just really tired. And apparently, later on, I was dropping off in between contractions and had a tiny micronap, so I felt like contractions were just constantly coming at me but it was because I'd fallen asleep in between.

Friend 1: I did that with my first baby and it was amazing… I didn't properly fall asleep, just sort of spaced-out, a twilight feeling. But then with my second, every time I fell asleep the contractions started. Which was fine, in terms of getting excited that they were starting again, but because I was so tired, from not being able to sleep, as soon as I was contracting all over the place, it felt like some sort of… I don't know…

Friend 2: Cruel trick.

Friend 1: Yeah… So would you have done anything differently if you could do the same labour again?

Friend 2: I don't think so. I think I probably did have the right level of help and intervention from the midwives in the end. I think the Pethidine did help because I was… Struggling, I suppose. They said, "It seems like you're having a tough time. Would you like some Pethidine?" But I hadn't thought to ask for it!

The pushing bit wasn't *as* awful… Well, actually, it was horrible, wasn't it?! But it wasn't as awful as I'd anticipated because that bit was actually quite quick. I think I was only pushing for about twenty minutes. So I was pleased that that was okay.

I was quite surprised at one point. They came and checked me and said I was only 4cm dilated. I was like, "Urgh, is that *all?!*" And they were like, "No, no, you're doing really well! We'll be back in four hours!" And I was like, "FOUR HOURS?! I'm so bored! You're just going to leave me for that long?"

Friend 1: I didn't know how much time had passed at all. The whole time. Turns out I'd been pushing for an hour with my first before someone came in and said, "That's enough now." But it didn't feel like an hour – it simultaneously felt like forever and about ten seconds.

Friend 2: I think I started pushing and then my contractions seemed to fade away a little bit, so they gave me some… No, no, again, they were going to give me something to bring the contractions on again but then I just pushed really *really* hard. So I was quite pleased that I managed to avoid that. I had a line in the top of my hand for most of the way through and things *nearly* kept needing doing and then they didn't, so that was quite nice. They gave me something to stop me feeling sick. I had (it must have been something with the Pethidine) to stop me feeling sick and that was it but yeah, I didn't need any of the inducing things.

Friend 1: What was your birth partner like?

Friend 2: He was brilliant! He didn't complain about being tired, even though he must have been absolutely knackered…

Friend 1: That's the thing that I didn't factor in at all with labour and it didn't hit me until about week 37 was… The realisation that I could go into labour at any point and it's going to be like running a marathon, but *I didn't know when it was going to start!* And I was probably going to have had no sleep because pregnancy sleeping is hard.

Friend 2: Ha! No, my birth partner was good – he'd been at work all day, and then he got home, and then I was like, "We *really* should go to Mothercare and make sure that the car seat's in properly. Can we definitely do that today? At some unreasonable time?" So we did that, then we got home, then two hours later my waters broke… So it was a good thing we did do that on that day!

Friend 1: Were you one day late? From your due date?

Friend 2: Yeah, one or two days, something like that. So pretty much on time.

Friend 1: I remember being really disappointed that your due date had gone. "You're meant to give birth on your due date! It's the date!"

Friend 2: "I want to see a baby!" Ha! I think I was probably sort of in denial about the whole "giving birth" thing right up to when it actually started happening. Like, that I would actually have to *have* the baby. Out of my vagina. Because that just doesn't seem like a good plan. Still. At my final midwife check, I was like, "So is this the one where you tell me that there's another way? That doesn't involve my vagina being ruined forever or major surgery?"

Friend 1: Ha! My vagina's actually fine now, fun fact.

Friend 2: Is it? After birth?

Friend 1: One of the things that haunted my labour was caused by a conversation I'd had just before, when a relative told me about her friend who'd had a 10lb baby. And the conversation went something along the lines of, "Can you imagine her fanny now? It must be like a bucket!" A bucket fanny. So then when *I* had a heavier baby, I thought, "This is it. Game over. It's going to be like the Channel Tunnel and strangers are accidentally going to end up walking right up in there." But then afterwards, I had some stitches and, honest to god, it was like a designer vagina. Totally ridiculous! The first time we had sex again after giving birth I was genuinely worried about how he was going to fit, i.e. totally the opposite of what I'd expected.

Friend 2: I didn't need any stitches.

Friend 1: You didn't need *any* stitches?!

Friend 2: Well, I grazed my labia, apparently, so I had a couple of stitches there, but the rest was fine.

Friend 1: Oh my god, I had *so* many!

Friend 2: I wanted to try having sex before my six-week check to make sure that it was basically fine… It was okay… But then at least two or three months after it was still… Not *painful*, but something wasn't right. Gosh, this sounds really bad, but it wasn't bad enough to stop (I was enjoying myself!) but it was still, at the beginning, just not quite right. It was *uncomfortable*. The first inch was sore and then the rest was fine. I had my smear and asked, "Can you just check if everything's alright?" And they said, "Yeah, it's a little bit inflamed," and sent off a swab, which was fine, and it just eventually got better. So I don't really know what the problem was. I guess the problem was that I'd had a baby! But yes, that's all over now. Phew!

Friend 1: One of the most painful things that happened to me after labour… I had external and internal stitches and the midwife, when she came to the house, asked if I'd like my stitches checked. I agreed and then she put (totally accidentally because she didn't know where they were) a finger *straight* on them. I thought my bits were on fire! She seemed so embarrassed and was very apologetic, and she'd been so gentle, it was just *quite* a sore place!

Friend 2: Yes, I bet.

Friend 1: So, speaking of stitches, I had an episiotomy…

Friend 2: Oh no!

Friend 1: No no no, I tore with my second and an episiotomy is *vay* better!

Friend 2: That's what I was really worried about.

Friend 1: So yeah, another fun fact, you can tear frontwards as well as backwards. Exciting! That was news to me!

Friend 2: Oooh! Overall, I feel like I escaped quite lightly. I *was* really worried about tearing. That's one of the things I said *as* she was coming out, *"I don't want to tear!"* And they said, "You won't!" and I said, "How do you know? You can't say that!" I guess it's either happened or it hasn't happened.

Friend 1: Before I had my first, I was thinking about labour and talking with women about their births and my approach, unsurprisingly, was, "Just tell me everything about it!" Virtually *everyone* said that stitches were an unexpectedly painful part of the process, especially if they hadn't had pain relief. You know, you think you've done it all, popped a baby out, and then it's, "*Now* you have to birth the placenta! And *now* you have to have some stitches!"

Friend 2: Do you think you would have done it differently with your first had you known his size? Did they recommend you have a C-section?

Friend 1: No, no. He wasn't clocked as big. He was, "SURPRISE! SUPER HEAVYWEIGHT!" And that was fine. With my second, in hindsight, I wish… I do wish that I'd been offered a C-section. The labour itself, when it actually happened, was so bloody fast. Fifteen minutes, one big push, he's here. So that was great. Ish. But the long days of sporadic contracting leading up to it…

Friend 2: I can't imagine…

Friend 1: Were just beyond awful. I saw so many midwives and they gave me *that* look with an, "Oh, this does happen!"

Friend 2: "And unfortunately it's happening to you!"

Friend 1: "Go and have a nice walk…" If only Bump had measured a bit bigger! The line was, "You've delivered a big baby vaginally, so you can do it again." Unless he showed up as bigger, we were to proceed as "normal". And I was actually happy about this at the time… But, knowing what I know now… All those days of labour stopping and starting… I think I would've been really insistent about not going through that… But hindsight is a wonderful thing.

Friend 2: Maybe it's because the pros know about all of the other things that could happen.

Friend 1: I did enjoy asking the midwives about that actually… Especially the ones who'd had children. I loved asking if their children had arrived before or after they'd become a midwife. And for those who said, "After," some did say it was quite a stressful experience because they know about all the things that can go wrong.

Friend 2: Generally, with most things, I do think about all the different things that can go wrong, but I assume it'll be fine. And I was assuming it would probably be fine. Like, right up until it started and then I went, "Oh no! This thing has happened that wasn't on the plan!"

Friend 1: I know!

Friend 2: I don't think they even read my birth plan because they would've seen "water birth"... Overall, I was really pleased with the midwives who delivered her, they left me to it about the right amount – I didn't feel abandoned but also they weren't hovering the whole time. The heartbeat monitor strapped around me did keep falling off though. And I also had to keep running off to the loo, so that didn't help because I had to keep taking it off, dashing to the loo, and then coming back...

Friend 1: I got so annoyed with the monitor and it falling off. The midwife kept adjusting it during contractions, I don't know if they did the same to you...

Friend 2: Yeah. Maybe something was going on with the contractions but they all just kept falling off. The only thing I was a little bit... Not disappointed with exactly, but surprised about was that I'd been moving around for most of the time during labour and walking about... I think at one point I really wanted to lie down but I didn't like being up on the bed, so I just lay on the floor, on one of those pads. And I think it was the student midwife who said, "I'm not sure if I'm allowed to let you lie on the floor," and I was like, "I'm lying on the floor!"

Friend 1: "It's *my* labour!"

Friend 2: I didn't like being up high on the bed.

Friend 1: That's the moment when I panicked the most, when I was up on the bed and they took the bottom of the bed away. I'd been leaning over a birth ball since contractions started and found vertical positions the most comfortable but then I needed my waters breaking so was confined to the bed... The midwife suggested that gravity would help but I didn't really understand what they'd done to the bed by taking the end off. I just assumed that I had to hold myself up and that I was the only thing stopping me from falling off the end of the bed! The next day, my arms were so sore because I'd been doing one giant push-up for the whole pushing phase!

Friend 2: They had me deliver lying on my back on the bed. Everything I'd read said that this was exactly *not* what I should've been doing. And I think I sort of feebly said something along those lines, but they reassured me that it was fine. Possibly because they really needed to see what was going on? I don't know. Slightly disappointed that I wasn't standing or on all fours or something like that, after I'd been vertical for so long before that.

Friend 1: Did you do NCT?

Friend 2: No.

Friend 1: No, I didn't either.

Friend 2: Just yoga and read things online about what happens. They were quite good actually. Just things like a midwife talking about labour and what would happen... But I didn't do anything that "official" like NCT because yeah, I just figured it'd be fine!

Friend 1: Did you have any friends who'd had babies before? Who you spoke to about labour?

Friend 2: No, not really… No close friends that I see regularly anyway.

Friend 1: That was one thing that gave me loads of confidence… A friend saying, after I'd just run that half-marathon, that if I can run that distance, then I can give birth to a baby – it's about the same amount of effort! Quite a weird comparison…

Friend 2: I'd spoken to a friend a little bit as well but not in depth. More about babies than birth.

Friend 1: If you have another baby, will you do anything differently do you think?

Friend 2: Well… I felt like I really didn't get to decide a lot of what happened. It was just, "This is what's happening now!" because of how it started… I probably would ask if I could go in the consultant-led unit because it was so nice and the room was so nice and I felt really looked after. I hadn't visited it, but I had visited the midwife-led unit and those rooms were smaller and not as nice. So I'd be quite happy now that I know you can have a midwife-led birth in the consultant-led unit…

Friend 1: I felt like that whole thing was very *Bullseye* in Cambridge. Like, "Look at what you could have won!" The midwife-led unit was *amazing*. The birth pool looked like a big hot tub, the bed's a double so your partner can get on there with you, bars, balls, an iPod station… It was bloody ridiculous, like a hotel! And then, when I did the tour, they said they wouldn't bother showing us the delivery unit because it'll all probably be fine. And then, when the news was

roken that it was going to be an induction, I was told the unit was
/here I'd be and I was like, "Where's my big birth pool?!" Although
wasn't induced on the right ward because the induction ward was
all but, because I was already beyond 42 weeks, they weren't happy
/ith me waiting any longer in case I gave birth to an elephant…
Which kind of happened anyway! So I was on a ward with people
/ho were there because something was really quite wrong.

Friend 2: The hospitals near us are all change, so by the time we
.ave another one I'll probably have to go somewhere else. It's not
hat far, not, like, dangerously far away but it was only twenty
ninutes to the one where I went last time… So that's slightly
nnoying. I don't know if their consultant-led unit will be as nice as
he one we have here, which is brand new.

Friend 1: In some places I don't think you really get a choice… I
idn't in the Midlands. I was consultant-led with my first because of
he induction and then, because the placenta got stuck, where we
ve now, they wanted to manage that part to make sure it all came
ut okay, so I was consultant-led again. I was very grateful in the
nd… But I was so excited with my second that I managed to do
he first stage of labour at home, in the bath, and I lit a candle… It
ecame really clear when it was too painful though. Also, we'd just
ad the bathroom done, so I wasn't entirely sure I wanted to spoil
:… I was literally looking between contractions thinking, "This is
potless! I don't want to spoil it with gunk!" And I also had this
hought: "What happens if my waters break in the bath?! How will
know?!"

Friend 2: Maybe a bit of blood? Possibly? A little splodge?

Friend 1: That's a good name for a baby, ha!

Friend 2: Sometimes they don't go till, like, halfway through anyway...

Friend 1: I didn't feel them go with my second at all. I *think* it all came out together with the final push. So, in the post-labour haze, I was totally convinced that he'd been born in the amniotic sac. I envisaged him looking like one of those little alien egg toys from the '90s! But the midwife just looked very confused and it appeared I'd just made that up! I had them broken with my first though.

How did you feel when baby was born?

Friend 2: I was like, "Ooh, there's a baby, this is going to be nice and I'm glad that's finished!" But I didn't get that sort of "[*gasps*] I'm going to care and protect for this tiny baby for my entire life and die for her!" feeling. I was more like, "Ooh, the baby's here, I've been looking forward to this!" The maternal rush of love came later.

Friend 1: Did you know you were having a girl?

Friend 2: No, no. I don't remember this but my husband says that they kept referring to the baby as "He" the whole way through, so he was a bit annoyed that they'd said what it was, but apparently that's their habit, to say, "He". I wasn't bothered, it's not very nice to just say, "It."

Friend 1: Yeah, that's true. Or, "They." We said, "They," because we didn't find out the sex and people automatically went, "Oh my

God, are you having twins?!" When Husband told me the sex, that was a really nice moment… Did yours cut the cord?

Friend 2: Yes, I think so. Yes. And he got to have a little cuddle when I had my shower.

Friend 1: The shower was both the most welcome and the most terrifying thing. I just didn't know how much it was going to hurt. That's one of the things that I found really weird on both recovery wards that I ended up on, I was the only person who showered the entire duration of the stay.

Friend 2: There was an en-suite bathroom in the room where I gave birth, so I could have a shower there. Then they took me down to the midwife-led unit to go on the ward and I stayed overnight. I'm really pleased that I did in the end.

Friend 1: I think that makes a big difference.

Friend 2: Well, mostly because she started vomiting bloody mucous! The midwife was standing right next to me when she did it and she said, "That's normal, that's your blood, not hers." I definitely would've panicked if I'd just got home and my newborn started puking brown!

Friend 1: I think it helps with breastfeeding as well. And all those little things… Like when my baby got hiccoughs and (so embarrassing now) but I asked the midwife if this was normal and what I should do. And she was like, "… Put a cold key down his back?!"

Friend 2: It's funny but that's it, you just don't know what you're supposed to worry about! You've been reading about looking after a baby for ages but you still don't *actually* know what to do. I remember when she was crying, I picked her up, she was still crying, and I thought, "How long does she cry for before I call a midwife?!"

Friend 1: In Cambridge they didn't let the baby cry at all. Every time baby cried someone came over. It was quite awkward when I was on the ward on my own and I had to go to the toilet…

Friend 2: Yes! I thought, "Am I allowed to leave my baby? Will I get told off for leaving my baby unattended?" I contemplated wheeling her into the bathroom in that little plastic tub…

Friend 1: I told the midwife I was going to leave him while I went to the toilet and she said, "He'll be fine." I asked, "Will anybody steal him?" She replied, "Probably not."

Friend 2: Yes, the mums have already got one of their own!

Friend 1: At Worcester baby had a little security tag around his ankle. Like the ones they put on whisky bottles in the supermarket! And they advised not to take a baby beyond a certain point without telling someone otherwise a massive security guard would wrestle you to the ground!

… I feel like there should be some sort of closing question to round things off apart from, "So it was okay then?"

Friend 2: It was alright, yeah! I think my overall impression was mostly that I was quite relieved that it was okay.

Friend 1: Yes, that's a question – was labour better than you thought it was going to be?

Friend 2: It was better than I'd feared but maybe not quite as perfect as I'd hoped.

Birth Journey M

When I imagined myself giving birth, I envisaged whale song, mood lighting, an inviting birthing pool, and simply to wander around a gorgeous birthing suite while my labour slowly progressed. Sadly, the birthing gods were not on my side and the reality was somewhat different.

My labour had to be induced three weeks early due to a multitude of problems but, in all honesty, having experienced a pretty horrific pregnancy (hyperemesis gravidarum, gestational diabetes, pelvic girdle pain… The whole shebang), I welcomed the decision with open arms. After three long, dull days of waiting for my labour to be started by pessary, and on the verge of losing my sanity having shared a ward with rude, noisy people, I was finally taken down to the delivery suite.

Being a chemical-free, zero-waste-shopping, henna-wearing, prayer-flag-hanging hippy, I was adamant that I didn't want any pain relief during labour. Not so I could be a hero, but purely because I had tried tremendously hard during pregnancy to live as "non-toxic" and "chemical-free" a lifestyle as possible. By the end of the three days of early labour, I'd managed to survive with no more than one injection of Pethidine (and that was purely so I could get some sleep between contractions). In the delivery suite, because labour was progressing so quickly, there wasn't time for anything "substantial" like an epidural... But I thought I could get through without one anyway. I liked knowing that each contraction was one step closer to ending this pregnancy.

Shortly after arrival to delivery suite, my waters were broken and a hormone drip inserted. My partner arranged our belongings neatly on the shelf and nested in his chair as I lay down and just kept thinking about how much I wanted a pizza, followed by the biggest nap in history. We were expecting many hours of waiting around before *The Big Show* started.

Within an hour, I had dilated to 5cm. Clearly my body was as ready to get this baby out as my brain was! After two hours, I was fully dilated and ready to push. Of course, the midwives told me that I was probably wrong – "Most ladies take much longer with their first babies" – but I climbed onto all fours regardless because I knew what my body was telling me to do. After a quick check on the "beepy machine", I was attached to many wires and dangly things and the midwife confirmed that I was, indeed, ready to push.

By the time she'd done this, I'd already experienced what most pregnant women hope to avoid. My bowels seemed to be *continuously* opening, thus requiring the poor student midwife to remain near my backside with a blue towel, wiping away my dignity plop by plop. I was waving my bottom around in the air like a hippo trying to attract a mate. The noises I was making with every contraction could probably be used in a Peruvian rain dance. In sum, I was a complete hot mess and I didn't care at all. I wanted it all to end. I wasn't excited, I wasn't happy, I wasn't ready.

They quickly gave me the gas and air so that I could get through pushing without making any more donkey noises or growls... This helped substantially. The staff were amazed that I didn't vomit after consuming so much of it! I pushed and pushed and pushed until I turned blue, had veins popping out of my neck, and thought I was going to push this baby out with such velocity that it would hit the wall. Unfortunately for me, it was no good. I had twisted myself into *every* position you could think of on that hospital bed until, eventually, they settled on the most undignified for me – on my back with my chubby little legs in stirrups. Whilst pushing, the pain in my lower back was worse than it had been during contractions. It was a deep, sharp, all-consuming pain that made me wish they could suck the baby out with a vacuum cleaner. Then, the dreaded words, "We're going to need to make a cut," were spoken… An episiotomy. At this stage, I didn't care if they cut off my legs, arms, or head; I just wanted it to end. They asked my permission, so I shouted, "YES, FINE! DO IT!", at which point the sweet student midwife calmly told me that they have to ask permission before they can do anything, to which I politely replied, "I understand completely but please just make it stop!"

As the baby was crowning, they asked if I wanted to feel the top of my baby's head. "Do I hell?!" I thought. "Why would I want to delay this any further?!"

In the end, I had a second-degree tear and they used a little suction cup on my son's head to help ease him out. Of course, they placed him straight on my chest for some skin-to-skin contact, while my partner was in floods of tears of both joy and horror. It's at this point that I'd love to be able to say that I was overcome with happiness and relief, however, I can't. They were practically doing press-ups on my stomach to force out the afterbirth that was taking a bit too long to come out. When it finally did come splashing out though, I felt the most incredible relief. More so than when the baby came out! It felt as though I'd lost half my body weight. This was the one and only positive thing that I can remember.

The anaesthetic they'd used while I was being sewn up hadn't taken effect. After a second sharp injection, it still didn't work. So I had to be stitched back together while on gas and air and I felt everything. Not quite the post-birth feeling I'd been expecting. This was shortly followed by a midwife coming running into the room and asking if I wanted to see my placenta. Does a cancer patient want to see their tumour? Do people want to see their appendix after it's been removed? Well, apparently, I had a very rare placenta. The umbilical cord fed directly into my major blood vessels, meaning that when my waters were broken, if the hook had been placed a centimetre or two to the right or left, I could have experienced mass blood loss requiring emergency surgery and/or a blood transfusion. Awesome. Thanks, Mother Nature. My partner still has the photographs of my magical, rare placenta... Not one for the mantelpiece I feel.

After four hours of quick but intensely painful labour, exhaustion had taken over. I held my son but couldn't quite comprehend that he was my child (the Entonox might have had a little something to do with that though). As awful as it sounds, at that moment in time, I still saw him as the cause of so much suffering and pain. All I wanted to do was sleep. I could hardly keep my eyes open and I felt like I couldn't hold up my own body weight, let alone a baby. I was dripping so much blood it was like someone had burst a blood bag between my legs. The overwhelming feeling of love for my newborn son had not reached me yet. All I wanted was to have a bath, put on some clean clothes, roll over, and sleep the days away.

Compared to what some women go through, my birth was not dramatic or full or terror, but to me, it was. I look back on it as a traumatic experience that I never want to repeat.

In hindsight, having cursed Mother Nature for being so cruel to me by gifting a horrific pregnancy and awful birthing experience, we are now friends again. She has blessed me with the most calm, clever, kind-natured, and hilariously funny little boy I could have ever hoped for and I'm eternally thankful… But I'm not in a rush to do any of it again!

Birth Journey N

My pregnancy was great – I felt fine (barely even pregnant, except for the lack of stomach muscles!) and I often joked that my labour would make up for it…

At 39 weeks of pregnancy, I was still only measuring 35cm and was sent for a growth scan. I started worrying when a friend said that they'd been induced the same day after a growth scan when baby was measuring small.

In for the growth scan, no concerns, 7lb 5oz baby predicted.

The staff said that I *might* not be allowed in the birth centre and this was gutting as I'd ideally wanted a water birth. But, at this stage, I was still down and planned for a birth-centre delivery.

My birth plan was to receive as little pain relief and intervention as possible but, if the midwives felt I needed anything, I'd take whatever was suggested.

At ten days overdue, I had my second sweep to try and encourage baby's arrival, had dinner out, and went to bed with mild backache. Throughout the night the back pain came and went, and at 3am it was a bit worse, so I got up for a wee and took some paracetamol. On return to bed my husband asked if this was it. I brushed it off, saying it was just back pain and was only hours apart…

From then on, I had contractions every two minutes lasting about a minute each. The contractions were really intense and still in my back. We rang the hospital who said I had ages and advised to get in the bath and relax. They said the pain would get worse as

I could still talk through the contractions. I got in the bath but needed to be on all fours due to the pain… And then I was sick. We called my mum (who was coming with us for the birth) and, when she arrived, she said we needed to get to hospital as I looked fairly progressed. We rang again and they agreed for me to go in. I had no idea how I was going to manage getting out of the bath, getting dressed, and a thirty-minute car journey!

I was sick again in the car and my husband wanted to stop to empty the bowl… But he was under strict orders – Do. Not. Stop. The. Car!

We made it into the ward and I felt like I needed the loo, where I then had another contraction. The midwife asked if I felt like I needed to push but I had no idea what that was supposed to feel like. They then assessed me and said I was 10cm dilated and should start pushing. I was glad – the pain was so bad that I don't think I would've coped if they'd said I was still in early labour! They got me on my side and I started pushing. But as they measured me (still small) and checked baby's heartbeat, they began to worry as it was dropping.

I was whisked to the delivery unit as they were worried about baby's slow heart rate and we were told that baby needed to be out in ten minutes. They gave me an episiotomy and a doctor was called for a forceps delivery. I delivered my baby before the doctor returned with the forceps! But then time stood still.

My baby was born in the sac (i.e. the waters never broke) with his cord wrapped tightly around his neck two times. He wasn't breathing. The midwife ripped open the sac, cut the cord, and passed the baby over to about eight people who were waiting, with all the arrest bells ringing. They ventilated him immediately and started inserting lines and tubes. After nine minutes, he finally took a breath and they picked him up and ran with him to NICU.

My mum, husband, and I were all in shock and just stood watching. We remember the midwife asking how he was doing. The reply was a shaking head, "Not good," and saying his oxygen levels were 7 so we needed to go up on the oxygen. The reply was that he was already on 100%. We were told that it'd be three hours before we could see him while they did tests and inserted more lines.

I was stitched up, had a drink, and we started to inform family. The rest of that day was a bit of a blur. Only two people at a time were allowed to see him and I was wheeled in. He was breathing on his own, in a cooling jacket to protect his organs, and had lines everywhere. He looked startled.

I went up to the ward where I would be admitted and complained of left shoulder pain and some epigastric pain. I was sick and Doctor said he needed to do some tests. My husband was allowed to stay overnight, so we tried to get some sleep. Doctors returned around midnight and said that I had preeclampsia. (They'd previously said that they were running tests for it due to my symptoms but thought I looked too well to have it. Turns out my blood pressure was 190 systolic and my liver function was abnormal. I still had negative urine dip though and none of the typical symptoms, such as headaches, blurred vision, and swollen hands and feet. And I didn't have any risk factors for preeclampsia either.) So I was taken to a close-observation unit for a catheter, put on "nil by mouth", hooked to a magnesium drip, and had my blood pressure checked every fifteen minutes.

My husband slept through this whole process but, after seeing me in labour, this was nothing.

The worst part was not being able to visit my son for the twenty-four hours that I was on bed rest. However, at 23:00 the following night, the nurses kindly took me on the bed to visit my son. They think I had undiagnosed preeclampsia late in pregnancy and that was why my baby only weighed 5lb 5oz. The fact he was so underweight meant that he didn't cope well with a fast (three and a half hours) and traumatic labour.

I improved and was moved back to a normal ward. We were given a private room, which was great; I didn't have my baby with me so the last thing I wanted was to be around other people's babies.

After three days, they slowly warmed my son up, a process that was slightly delayed as he experienced a couple of seizures, which they said is common. They said that once the cooling jacket was off, we could hold him… But I had to wait until he was four days old. The nurse passed him to me and I was able to hold him for an hour. He still had lots of lines and attachments. I was expressing milk and he was fed this through a nasal tube.

We were gradually able to get more involved in changing nappies, dressing him, and giving him his milk. He was one week old before my husband was able to hold him. Our baby was moved to a lower-dependency bay but was then moved back as his oxygen levels were dropping. I was told I could go home but I refused to leave hospital without my baby. Luckily, I was able to stay for another two days as the bed wasn't needed and then NICU arranged accommodation on site for me. Over those few days I don't think I ever stopped crying.

My son had an MRI scan and we were told he had a brain injury from lack of oxygen during birth. This meant he was either absolutely fine, or severely disabled, and we would only know the outcome as he grew and developed. Not knowing was horrible. You just want answers… Will he be okay? When can we go home? Other parents and the hospital staff were so supportive and thankfully we had lots of family support too.

Eventually, we were allowed to hold him more often and I started trying to breastfeed, before we finally moved to the ward where I could stay with him. Baby fed every three hours for twenty-four hours, his nasal feeding tube came out, and we were allowed home.

We've had regular follow ups since – initially every two months, then five months, and now nine – and they're really happy with his progress. Normally I wouldn't say I'm a worrier, but I've been so desperate for him to be able to do everything that it's been hard when other babies have beaten him to it. Even though there's a wide range of "normal" and he did some things before other babies!

I honestly believe that if we hadn't been in hospital when I gave birth, then my son wouldn't be alive. We owe that to the amazing hospital team.

I think we've felt every emotion along the way… Guilt if we did something that made him poorly, like travel vaccinations, dietary changes, horse-riding… Lucky that we're fortunate to have a gorgeous son who's healthy and that we were able to bring him home relatively early compared to some families… Misfortune that we should be the ones to experience all this trauma when other people have fairly routine labours and healthy babies… Grief for missing out on skin-to-skin, newborn cuddles, and the routine post-labour experience.

No-one can ever truly understand that NICU experience unless you've been there yourself. There are still parts of our journey that make me cry but, luckily, our story has a happy ending.

For anyone in a similar position, do contact this book's editor for my details. It definitely helps to talk about these things and I'm happy to help... I promise that it does get easier.

Birth Journey O

After Baby tricked us with a false labour amid the "Fryken and Svartsjön" of an Ikea bathroom display at 32 weeks, my real contractions began at 40 weeks and 3 days. I'd had some slight cramps and twinges for a couple of days and had found our evening walk, in the sweltering heat of an Indian Summer, up Telegraph Hill more like a trek up Kilimanjaro. I didn't feel anything in particular before going to bed but woke up at 02:00 with strong, period-pain-like cramps. I decided not to wake up the papa-to-be but got up, had a walk about and some water, and remembered that this most probably was far from delivery, and so went back to bed and slept. At 06:00, I finally cracked and woke up my partner and told him to take the day off work. At 08:00, we called the maternity unit and spoke to a midwife who, as predicted, told us my contractions needed to be at least "one in five" before we could come in. Mine were about one in every twelve minutes.

Having checked The Bag a few times, we decided it would be best to crack on with the day, so off we went to the post office. The lady at the counter asked when I was due.

"Now," I told her.

"NOW?!"

She responded with a look of terror in her eyes, before wishing us luck.

Our next stop was Sainsbury's, with me continuously stopping and leaning on the papa-to-be so that I could breathe, try and remember hypnobirthing techniques, and curse myself for not having been more regimental in practising them.

At about 19:00, we thought contractions reasonably close enough together and hypnobirthing-techniques-going-out-of-the-window enough to make our way to the hospital. After a quick examination, I was told, disbelievingly, that I was ZERO centimetres dilated. And that I needed to be at least 4cm to be taken seriously. I felt rather disappointed in myself – how could this be? I'd been at it since 02:00!

Home we went.

As the pain increased while at home, I decided the best place to be was in the bath with a continuous flow of warm water and the comforting mumbles of Radio 4. The papa-to-be bedded down in the bathroom doorway to sleep. Having listened to episodes of *The Archers* since the beginning of time, I found my contractions intensifying and the bath was feeling too small to contain us. Feeling the pain more desperately and my contractions moving closer together, we decided to go to the hospital again…

"Surely this is it now! I must be at least 4cm!"

Having already been in once, I was worried we would be turned back again but, as we stood on the street corner by the hospital, breathing through a contraction, an old lady with the most perfect afro appeared. She told me how well I was doing, how everything was going to be fine… She then explained that she was a midwife just coming off her shift and that she would see me tomorrow to deliver our baby. There was something mystical about her and she really put me at ease.

We carried on into the hospital where, on examination, I was told I was 1cm dilated. ONE CENTIMETRE! How could this be?! I felt like crying. I was finding the pain hard to bear and the midwife suggested Pethidine to relieve it. I swiftly replied with a "Hell, no!" We'd decided against using Pethidine after reading up on it in our NCT course. Asked, "Why?" I couldn't remember, I just knew it was bad. After the midwife explained The Negatives (which did then ring a bell), she explained that I was so far off delivery that it would do no harm, so I backed down and agreed. The injection meant that I could not go home but I was given a bay in the pre-labour ward. Being surrounded by blue curtain with a distinctly clinical atmosphere was not part of "The Plan", but I held on to mindfulness and that I would eventually get to 5cm and that I would eventually get to the midwife-led suite… "The Plan".

The Pethidine seemed to do nothing for me and my contractions became stronger and stronger; they felt like the worst period pain (for me that means great pain in my lower back and feeling like I'll lose the ability to walk). Thankfully, at this point, the midwife was able to hook me up to some gas and air, which came as a great relief.

Somewhere along the line, I thought my waters had broken as my mucous plug passed on a trip to the loo – surely this must be it now! Having proudly declared to the midwife that my waters had broken, on later inspection I was told that, in fact, no, they had not. This experience now felt like forever. I was extremely tired and becoming increasingly emotional and irritable. While the gas and air was helping with the pain, I started to feel like I was never going to get to the midwife-led unit and didn't feel like I could give birth in my current surroundings. I wanted to get out of there. I told the midwife that I couldn't take it anymore. Assuming I was talking about the pain, she told me that I could not have an epidural. At this I snapped, "It's not the plan!" I believe this prompted the midwife to read my birth plan for the first time. I just wanted to be in water again.

Shortly afterwards, a kind midwife told us we could go up to the unit but that we needed to take the stairs. Looking back, I assume this was an attempt to get me more dilated as I still wasn't quite there yet. As we made our way down the corridor, I felt like my ass was going to fall out. So much pressure was pushing down I was convinced I was going to prolapse there and then in the corridor as I held onto the handrail and squatted down with a contraction. There was no way I would make it up the stairs without my ass falling out!

We got a wheelchair and went up to the midwife-led suite. As we entered, the lady with the beautiful afro welcomed us. I realised it must be the next day. Again, she put me at ease. Seeing the birthing pool, I practically tore my clothes off and jumped straight in. The water was so soothing and I could have gas and air on the side. We made ourselves at home, put music on, ate dates and apricots, and enjoyed the water. It felt luxurious compared to minutes ago. Unfortunately, our guardian angel's shift ended but we were blessed with another midwife and student midwife who respected our request for minimal intervention and left us to it in a calm atmosphere.

Another shift came and went… I was dilating so slowly. Papa-To-Be started to suffer from sleep deprivation and dehydration, so took a nap on the bed while I stayed in the birthing pool with the new midwife and student midwife looking after me, again with the most respect and calm. Eventually, we realised that I hadn't peed for a long time and this could be a reason why things were moving so slowly; my bladder was blocking the baby and the baby was blocking my bladder. I agreed to a catheter and had a record-breaking wee.

Back in the pool and, well and truly pruned, I suddenly felt the urge to get out of the water and knelt by the side of the bed with a beanbag. I was so tired, I wanted to sleep, but Papa-To-Be and the midwives urged me on. I started to feel a bit claustrophobic and told everyone to back off. I needed a few minutes to refocus and then, despite the lingering memory of my anthropology professor punching his fist through a model pelvis to demonstrate what happens when you give birth on your back, I felt that this exact position was where I would be most comfortable at this point... Able to see my surroundings and the people with me.

Soon, the urge to push became so strong. After two or three big contractions, the midwife said I could put my hand down and feel the baby's head. For me, that was a big turn off, I didn't want to, I just wanted to see and hold our baby. One more big contraction and there Baby was, with me, on my chest, so squashed and slippery. I had an inkling that Baby would be a boy, but nobody did The Big Reveal and, as his name settled in my mind, I had to ask. I was too scared to lift him to see for myself, worried I would drop my precious bundle. A boy, I held him close and kept his name to myself for the moment.

At this point, the focus went from Baby to delivering the placenta. I started to feel a little anxious as I had foolishly read some horror story about a uterus that had inverted during the process. Perhaps because of this delightful recall, I was a little tense and it seemed difficult to deliver the placenta. After having an injection and some encouragement from the midwife, all seemed to be well, and the placenta was taken off for inspection and the umbilical cord for donation. The midwife informed me that I had torn a little after all and would need stitches. After reassuring me about the extent of the tear, it became apparent that I was bleeding quite badly, and an emergency team appeared out of nowhere. Papa held our son while the anaesthetist explained the situation. I didn't really feel scared until I thought, "Maybe I'm not scared because I'm dying and they're just not telling me," so I decided to ask. Upon being reassured that I was not about to die, I felt at ease and full of love. Slowly the emergency team disappeared as my bleed came under control and the midwife was left to sew me up. At this point, I asked what day it was. I realised it was now, in fact, my birthday and loudly hoped that the midwife would do her best with the stitches. Delirious with love for the world and with sleep deprivation, I was cracking jokes all over the place. I'm not sure if it was my oxytocin high or the effect of so much gas and air, but I felt on top of the world!

Finally, at 05:00, we left the birthing suite and were given a bed in the postnatal ward. We were welcomed by a chorus of snores. We waved goodbye to the midwives and settled down for some sleep, one eye half-open, gazing at our son. It felt unreal – he was finally here, safe and sound. I'd had simply the best birthday gift, stitches and all.

Birth Journeys P, Q & R

My first pregnancy was wonderful... I loved being pregnant! I had never felt so fulfilled and I had very little morning sickness. I got tired more easily but I felt fantastic! Like every first-time mum, I was so excited at the prospect of my baby's arrival. In all honesty, as the day drew closer, I also felt quite frightened. I had read all the books but I still didn't feel *prepared*.

Looking back, I think it was a confidence thing. Everyone I came into contact with had done their job so many times that it was all so ordinary to them. I suppose that was, in some ways, reassuring, but not everyone was the ideal midwife or doctor... Sometimes I felt like an object.

I had read so much about being able to make all these choices. In reality, however, I felt as though I had to fit *their* mould. The "choice" of a C-section was the last thing I wanted but, by that point, I knew there was no other option. My husband was so brave. Whilst they kitted him out with scrubs, I held onto a trainee midwife to try to stay still enough between contractions so that I could have the spinal inserted. She was an angel, keeping calm, and so down to earth, which kept me calmer too. Being awake during the birth was awesome! Suddenly, from nowhere, this baby was put into my arms.

My experience was not a bad one and I delivered a healthy baby via emergency section eleven days over my due date. After thirty-five hours of labour and an emergency section, I was physically exhausted and mentally shell-shocked. My 9lb 1oz baby girl was beautiful and precious. I was quite overwhelmed by the entire experience, which had not gone according to any of the plans I had in mind!

*

Baby Number Two came seventeen months later. I felt a little more relaxed about this birth because I had been through the whole thing before. However, there was still a latent fear that this birth would not be easy. Would this turn into another C-section or would this be a "normal" delivery? As it turned out, this beautiful 9lb baby girl was longer and thinner with a smaller head! The midwife was a more experienced lady who acted with complete conviction and had a very reassuring air. She had no doubts about whether this baby would be a "normal" birth… And she was right! I felt more relaxed in her care than I had in that of my previous lady. The midwife knew exactly what she was doing and this helped me so much.

The birth did leave me with little red blood spots all over my body… One minute there was talk of needing a blood transfusion, the next I was being sent home. I felt as weak as a kitten, but happy. It was very tiring having two little ones to care for, but I think I had found my niche in life… I just loved being a mum.

*

My son was born ten years later. He was a healthy 8lb 15 oz. I had concerns about being an older mother but my consultant and all other staff kept reassuring me that this was no problem because

I was fit and well. Although this birth was the most recent, it is the one I remember least well. My main recollection is that, at one point, I felt as though I had the entire maternity staff in my room watching what was going on! It was a bit of a circus. They even made my husband a sandwich during all the commotion!

The delivery was relatively straightforward and I felt pretty calm throughout. The most difficult part of this pregnancy and birth had occurred in the earlier stages. A test was recommended that involved a long needle being inserted through my stomach and into the placenta to get a sample of my baby's DNA. My husband and I travelled down to King's College Hospital in London. I had the test done under local anaesthetic and then went home. Although the staff were very good, I was just another routine procedure and no-one took the time to reassure me. I wasn't told to take things easy, so I just continued with my life as normal. When the pains began the next day, I truly believed that I was going to miscarry this baby. I drove myself home in a blind panic. When I read the leaflets thoroughly, I found out about the risks, as well as the recommendations for taking things easy for a day or so. As it turned out, my body was just moaning about having that huge needle inserted! Who can blame it for that? When the results came through and it was all clear... What a relief!

*

The NHS provided me with excellent midwives, health visitors, GPs, and consultants. They were all over-worked but the majority of them were there because they love what they do. And I thank every last one of them for that.

Birth Journey S

They tell you when you're pregnant that your waters won't break like they do in the movies; that there's no big dramatic torrent. Mine did. With it came a surge of relief and emotion like I've never felt in my life.

My labour had started a few days earlier and, after being in and out of hospital, I was waiting it out patiently at home with frustratingly slow contractions. On the Tuesday evening, I had concerns about reduced foetal movement, so we went to hospital to be checked. Thankfully, all was well, but as this was our second episode of reduced movement, we were told I was to be admitted to hospital and induced that night. I was several days overdue by this point and, although an induction wasn't what I wanted, I was happy at the thought of getting on with things so we could finally meet our baby.

Unfortunately, circumstances were not on our side. We were amongst several others who were admitted that night, all of whom had higher-risk deliveries than I did. The induction ward was overwhelmed with women needing this intervention. Over the following forty-eight hours I lived and breathed the full force of the staffing and resource shortages currently facing the National Health Service. Delivery rooms were available but there were not enough midwives, and the pressure they faced compromised their care and compassion.

A couple of times a day I was hooked up to a machine that monitored our baby's heartbeat and was supposedly measuring my contractions. The machine was connected to a central computer at the midwives' desk outside the room. This information was being used to prioritise us in the induction queue. The machine was missing at least half of my contractions and the remoteness of the staff meant that they were missing the very obvious visual clues that I was having a contraction. When I questioned what was going on and said I was contracting as much as I was, I was dismissed and ignored.

At one point, to try and ease the pressure on the ward, they tried to move me to a nearby hospital with a poor reputation, which would have meant transferring me there in a taxi, in rush hour, in the rain, on a notoriously congested stretch of road (my partner was so sleep-deprived that he didn't feel safe driving me). We refused the transfer. My partner ended up insisting that a midwife came and sat by my side to monitor my contractions, so that they could be compared with those picked up by the machine. They eventually conceded that I was further along than they believed. I also insisted on a vaginal examination. I was clearly beyond 4cm dilated and so was technically in active labour. Yet still we waited.

All this time we were very concerned for our baby's wellbeing. Having been admitted to hospital because I *needed* to be induced *that same night* and then left to wait for so long was baffling. We fully respect that there were urgent cases that needed attention before us but the total lack of engagement, empathy, and support from the staff on the induction ward was making things so much worse for us. They admitted they didn't believe how far along I was because, when they did see me, I appeared to be coping. I'd done pregnancy yoga, which included learning a lot of breathing techniques for labour; while these were helping me to cope, they were also working against me by doing so, and I remained lower down in the queue than I should have been.

By the Thursday night, I was 6cm dilated and we were going out of our minds with sleep deprivation, pain, and worry. We'd resorted to speaking to another hospital who said that they had a space for me if we could get there. It was too late that night for a discharge but we resolved to leave first thing in the morning.

Thankfully, at just past midnight, my waters broke. We could escape the induction ward and head to the delivery unit.

I was half-asleep when my waters broke and, given the dramatic way in which they burst, both I and the bed were completely soaked. I was told to have a shower before going to the delivery unit and my partner ended up hosing me down while I was leaning against the wall, trying to breathe through some very strong contractions. From this point on, everything changed. The stress and worry seemed to wash away down the plughole... We were finally getting somewhere!

My birth plan had involved starting with gas and air and seeing how that went, but the previous few days had left me physically and emotionally exhausted before I was anywhere near the point of pushing. I agreed straight away to an epidural to help me cope, as well as the gas and air. I don't remember very much of what happened between then and when our baby was born; I was making the most of the effects of the gas and air, and using all the energy and cognitive power that I had left to get us through this last vital stage.

When it came to pushing, I managed to get our baby most of the way there but I didn't have the strength to finish the job. We were told that forceps were needed and, if they didn't work, an emergency caesarean. My partner had been handling everything amazingly but having to scrub up for theatre was when he started to struggle. Apparently, I told him to take a selfie in his scrubs… Obviously a priority at that point! I remember being moved to theatre and lots of buzzing activity… But I can't properly remember the actual moment of our baby's birth. This is still a very emotional issue for me. All I do remember is that I was getting frustrated – with my gown pushed up around my chest and with me lying flat on my back, I couldn't see her properly when she was handed to me.

We came home the day after the birth and had our first night together as a family. I was trying to breastfeed, it wasn't working well, and our baby was getting dehydrated and jaundiced. We ended up in Paediatric A&E and were admitted back into hospital. Sitting on a bed in A&E while medics repeatedly tried to get blood out of our two-day-old baby's heel was one of the worst experiences of my life. The previous week had taken such a toll on me that I barely managed to cope during the following few days in hospital. Thankfully, the amazing nurses on our ward took care of our baby at night so I could catch up on sleep and start to find my feet as a mother.

Birth plans often go out of the window; things can happen that aren't what you'd choose. The most important thing of all is that our daughter arrived safely. I know all that in my head… But, in my heart, I have an immense feeling of frustration and sadness that the stress and challenges of the days before my waters broke left me physically unable to deliver her without intervention or to remember fully the most important part of the whole experience. Worse still, I was in a terrible state for the first few days of our daughter's life. I felt like a failure as a mother when she needed me. It took a couple of weeks for that feeling to fade.

Induction, had it happened, may have resulted in a better or a worse experience. I will never know.

Birth Journey T

In the Beginning

"Oh God, I wish this wasn't happening!"

Not what I'd imagined I'd be thinking when my waters broke. It's around 04:00 on Friday, I'm in a hospital miles away from home, and I'm only 29 weeks pregnant.

*

We knew that there was a higher risk of premature birth with twins. Thanks to a one-day TAMBA (Twins and Multiple Birth Association) course, we'd been through what would happen if the babies were very premature, the weeks that we'd have ahead of us on a neonatal unit. I just didn't think it would happen to us. Up until this point, I'd had a very straightforward pregnancy – no morning sickness and no complications arising from having identical twins sharing a placenta.

I'd gone to the hospital after a few days of leaking fluid following what I suspected was the loss of my mucous plug. After several hours of having my "tightenings" monitored (none were registering as contractions), they finally examined me to discover I was 1cm dilated. I was told that either I might stay that way for a few weeks, or that the babies could be arriving right now. The hospital, however, had no neonatal cots left due to two sets of twins being delivered in the previous couple of days. Cue several hours of nurses trying to find me a hospital where I could be transferred. Mostly the response was, "Sorry, no room at the inn!"; nowhere had free both a delivery suite and the two neonatal cots required in specialist PICU (Paediatric Intensive Care Unit). It was 02:00 on Thursday before a hospital was found and I was promptly driven there in an ambulance, my husband speeding behind in our car.

I spent the day having on and off contractions at irregular intervals. A scan showed that the babies were both fine and "Twin 1", whom we had thus far named "Hiccup", was head down, meaning that a natural delivery was still on the cards. No-one really thought I was in labour; my contractions were still not registering. When I started shivering uncontrollably, the midwives on the ward didn't recognise that I was in shock. My body was pumping with adrenaline, preparing.

The contractions got worse through the night. I didn't get any sleep, my exhausted husband crashed out on a recliner chair next to me. I went to the bathroom… And my waters didn't so much break as *explode*, filling me with pure dread. What was going to happen? Were my babies going to be okay? I'd received two steroid injections to help mature their lungs, just in case. It takes twenty-four hours for them to be effective… It had been twenty-eight hours since I'd had the first one. That gave me a little solace.

I hadn't been examined since the night before as they didn't want to trigger my labour if it hadn't started yet. I was now a whopping great 9cm dilated! I wanted to go ahead with the natural delivery, if possible. The consultants were very supportive and seemed pretty relaxed. In fact, everyone seemed really calm (apart from us), so I felt like I was in good hands. After some manoeuvring of Hiccup to get a tiny hand away from their head and out of the way, we were good to go. I was now getting the uncontrollable need to push with the contractions and was moved to the delivery suite.

The consultant asked me about pain relief and if I wanted an epidural. We'd been told on the TAMBA course that hospitals want to give an epidural for a twin pregnancy because it's likely that the second baby will require a lot of manoeuvring. As I'd already had Hiccup moved around (unbelievably uncomfortable and unpleasant but not painful as such), they were okay with my refusal. The consultant said, "Well, you've coped fine so far, and you seem pretty relaxed, so okay, no epidural!" In the space of about twenty seconds, the decision had come and gone. I was pretty shocked that that was it and panicked that I'd just made a terrible decision.

*

Active Labour

I've spent a few hours with the midwife (one of two, the other's at a computer... I think... Typing notes? Monitoring the three of us?... She's a blur). My labour is now fully underway. In the midst of a contraction and pushing and inhaling gas and air, she tells me that it's now a shift change and that she's off...

WHAT THE HELL?!

In walks the most beautiful woman – my new midwife. I'm half-naked, sweaty, sleep-deprived, and this gorgeous young woman with immaculate make-up walks in.

"Hi! I'm Katy!" she says, far too sunnily for my mood. I barely say hello.

"Who the fuck?!" I think. "I don't care who you are! I want the other midwife back! I'm in the middle of active labour and you bound in all chipper and 'Nice to meet you!'" None of which I actually say out loud – I'm normally a nice person and fortunately still have functioning inner monologue. She seems like one of those millennials who are overly enthusiastic about everything. I feel like she should be serving me coffee in a way-too-trendy café in Shoreditch.

The pain of labour isn't what I've anticipated. The contractions are like period pain that just gets more and more intense, and just at the point where you can't bear it for a moment longer, it fades away. It's like a sea of discomfort building to a wave of incredible pain that washes over you… And then it's gone. What I wasn't expecting was the pain that came with the active labour. Not the ripping, tearing, agonising pain that I was expecting, but the pain of sheer physical effort. That pain of burning muscles that are screaming at you with the exertion. With it comes the focus you get in a major workout when you're pushing yourself to the limit. Just when you think you've given everything you have, when your muscles scream and you think you've got nothing left, your glamorous personal trainer Katy says to you, "Keep going, you're doing amazingly, push push push!" and you go for ten more seconds than you thought you had in you. Then you collapse back for a couple of minutes, maybe you fall asleep (didn't think that would be possible but that's exactly what I'm doing!) I'm in a zone of concentration, effort, burning, pushing, and pain. All I can hear is Katy, my focus is completely on her instructions and the pure physical exertion of my labour. Katy encourages me, guides me, tells me I'm doing amazingly, congratulates me after every round of pushing. She's transforming in front of me into my absolute hero.

I have only gas and air for pain relief and I'm not sure what helps more – the gas or having something in my mouth to bite down on. I don't know how my experience compares with birthing a larger baby. With small babies, there's not much to push against. They also don't do any of the work for you that a term baby might do to wriggle their way out to freedom. I'm pushing 100% actively on top of the involuntary pushes of my contractions. I'm certain that if I'd had the epidural, I would now not be able to get these babies out on my own.

Hiccup is on the way. A couple of consultants come in to see how things are progressing. I become aware that there's an entire team waiting outside the room – with two babies comes two of everything else... Two midwives, two obstetricians, two paediatricians, and goodness knows how many other doctors and nurses. It's like a Noah's ark of healthcare professionals! They start trickling in as I'm prostrate, naked from the waist down, and in the middle of a contraction. A few of them start setting up behind a screen to do... Well, whatever it is they're going to do when Hiccup arrives. One consultant tells me to make a fist and place it under the small of my back – an incredibly effective piece of advice, it must allow the pelvis to open. Very useful if you've ended up on your back rather than upright on a birthing ball, listening to peaceful music, and breathing through it all like you'd imagined. They decide to put my legs in stirrups and I don't care. I've gone from being unable to undress in a women's changing room to being almost naked with my legs up in stirrups in a room full of people. I'm amazed at how little this bothers me! As is my husband, who I think is far more alarmed by this than I am.

We're almost there...

There just isn't quite enough room for Hiccup to get out, so they're going to make a tiny cut. I'm virtually unaware of the multitude of injections they're giving me (anaesthetics, I assume). Katy makes a small cut (the doctors later marvel at the neat and tiny cut she's made and I'm grateful not to have had a gung-ho doctor go to town slicing me open!) I don't think the cut hurts, I think I'm just feeling the pressure of it. One more almighty push… And Hiccup is out!

"It's a girl!" Katy tells us. Immediately she's placed into a plastic sheet to keep her warm. My husband and I look at each other and burst into tears.

"Is she okay?" I ask. Katy nods at me, smiling. My daughter is placed into my lap for a few seconds so I can see her. She's so tiny! And then she's gone…

She's taken behind the screen and I don't really know what's happening in those first few moments of her life. My husband goes to see her while I catch my breath.

The moment Hiccup was born, the other midwife had put her hands on my stomach to catch "Twin 2" (also known as "Fidget") and stop her from going anywhere. Apparently, the second twin likes to stretch out and enjoy the space that's now left unoccupied by their sibling, which doesn't make their delivery particularly easy. It's barely been a couple of minutes… But the focus is now on the second delivery. Here we go again!

Fidget is breech, the consultant is going to have to help her out. This is uncomfortable and unnatural and unpleasant, but it's not unbearable. With the next contraction, her legs are out. They wait for the next contraction. When it comes, the consultant twists and pulls her… And she's out.

The same question – "Is she okay?"

She is.

*

The Aftermath

It's suddenly all over. Everyone leaves except Katy. My babies are whisked away to a neonatal unit and it will be four hours until I see them again, but I'm feeling incredible. I've done it! The sense of achievement is overwhelming – I've just brought two tiny people into the world. It seems very lonely and surreal now that it's just my husband and Katy in the room. They both tell me how amazingly I've done. Despite the circumstances, it was the best delivery I could have hoped for.

Katy brings me a cup of tea – it's the best damn tea I've had in my life! I've been "nil by mouth" since my waters broke, in case they needed to take me for surgery, so I haven't consumed anything other than a couple of energy gels since the night before. I'm showered and in fresh clothes when the paediatrician comes to see us. This conversation is the first we've had with anyone about the complications of having babies almost three months prematurely. He's mostly positive, there's a good chance they'll be perfectly normal, but we have a long road ahead... And not knowing what the future holds for our girls is terrifying.

We eventually get to see them on the neonatal unit. They're tiny – 2lb 9oz and 2lb 6oz – amongst a mass of wires for monitors and tubes for feeding. The unit is full of beeping equipment that will eventually haunt us in our sleep. We have so much love for them, but this environment is so alarming and alien.

Our journey is largely smooth sailing. After seven and a half weeks and three different hospitals (we're moved closer to home, hospital by hospital, until we're finally back in the hospital where I was meant to deliver), our tiny girls are allowed to come home. They slowly grow and we await their milestones with trepidation. Instead of the normal five- or six-week wait to see them smile, we wait sixteen – the world suddenly changes when they do. They hit every milestone, physically and developmentally. They are amazing. When their personalities start to come through, they are funny and cheeky and bright. We have just celebrated their second birthday and are incredibly thankful to have these two perfect little people in our lives.

Birth Journey U

As a busy working mum with a beautiful two-year-old daughter, I was so relieved when it was time to begin my maternity leave. I had been working shifts two nights a week and felt very tired and in need of some rest before the new baby arrived. My second baby was due on 21 January 1989 and we were so excited that our little family was going to be complete. Our closest friends (at that time) had moved away from where we had all grown up together, so the offer of a festive break in their new home sounded fantastic. Over Christmas and New Year, I felt very tired and a bit overwhelmed, but I just put it down to working too hard before the new baby's arrival.

We came home on 4 January and, by this time, I was feeling much more myself and had more energy to spend some quality time with my daughter. On 6 January I got up as usual and went to make my husband some sandwiches to take to work and *whoosh!* My waters broke! Oh no! This was way too soon! All sorts of emotions ran through me. This had been a much easier pregnancy than my first – no bleeds, no weight loss, no fainting, no low blood pressure – and I was much more confident second time around, physically and emotionally.

My husband worked in a bank. At that time fathers who already had a child at home were allowed two days' paternity leave. With my practical head on, I told my husband to go to work; I would go to the hospital (in an ambulance, as per my GP's instructions) and then phone the bank when I got there saying that my waters had broken and the baby was on its way. That way, 6 January did not have to count as one of his paternity leave days – genius!

By this point, even though my waters had broken, I did not have any contractions at all. I was admitted to hospital and I sat on the maternity ward all day. By late afternoon, still nothing. Visiting time came and went, and my husband went home. I can remember sitting in a side room on my own at teatime, eating the fish and chips that someone else had ordered from the hospital menu the day before, and wishing that something would happen and that my baby would be here. My vital signs were taken throughout the day and at 18:00, I was wired up to a monitoring machine to ensure that everything was progressing satisfactorily. By 18:30, the midwife checked the machine and decided that the baby was "stressed"; she was a little concerned. The duty doctor examined us and said it would be better if I went up to the delivery suite and I was "started", as he put it. Then things began to happen very *very* quickly!

I can remember asking for my husband (before the days of mobile phones) and the nursing assistant assured me that she would telephone him and that he would be there as soon as possible. I went up to the delivery suite. A doctor and midwife began to prep my hand for inserting a needle and drip into it whilst talking to each other about the night before (they'd been out somewhere socially). I was so afraid. Even though this was my second baby, things were very different here compared to when I'd had my first baby, and nobody was telling me anything. I felt like a piece of meat on a supermarket trolley that had to be sorted out and dealt with. I burst into tears (looking back, quite dramatically) as I was so scared.

"What's the matter?" the midwife asked.

"What are you doing to us?" I replied. "Why all the needles and drips?"

"Just a little something to get the contractions going…"

And boy, did they get going! It was only a matter of minutes before the first contraction came and it was very sharp and painful. Again, totally different to my first labour where the pain had built up gradually and slowly. The contractions seemed to go from 0-60 miles an hour within minutes, not hours. Thankfully, my husband soon appeared, all gowned up, and I have never been so pleased and relieved to see anyone in my entire life.

The consultant examined me at 20:20 and told my husband that I would be at least another *two hours* – he should go and get himself a cup of tea! I panicked at this advice as I knew I only had a very short time to go before needing to bear down and push.

"Don't leave me!" I shrieked at my husband and grabbed his arm so tightly that the next day he had a bruise!

Then, as happened during my first labour, I had to have an episiotomy. The scissors used were quite blunt and I saw my husband wince as they were changed for a sharper pair. To be honest, I was in so much pain by this stage, it all just melted into one big hurt. Luckily my husband didn't go anywhere and my baby was born twenty minutes later, at 20:40. Thank goodness he didn't take the advice given to him – he would have missed everything and I would have given birth on my own!

I was totally convinced my new baby was going to be a girl; there had not been a baby boy born to my side of the family since the late 1940s and scans taken in the 1980s did not reveal the sex of the baby to the parents (they were purely to spot any abnormalities or disabilities in order for you to make an informed choice). When the midwife exclaimed, "You have a beautiful baby boy!" I was actually speechless!

"What are you going to call him?" she asked.

"… Kathryn Victoria?!" came my reply. I hadn't even thought of any boys' names!

He weighed in at 8lbs 13.5oz. Phew! Thank goodness he had decided to come two weeks early, as goodness knows how large he would have been if we had made it to term!

Birth Journey V

The birth of our firstborn was started by induction. It's a surprisingly odd feeling to walk calmly into a hospital knowing that you'll leave with a child (your own child, preferably). In pregnancy, you prepare yourself for the 02:00 "My waters have broken!" moment, you've battle planned how you're going to get a labouring woman into the car, which route to the hospital will be the best to take depending on the time of day… You've strategized, you've packed bags with military precision (they are by the door – not so invasive that you're looking at them constantly, but close enough that you can grab them on the way past while supporting a birthing mother). The next thing we're told is that the induction is quite a slow process and that, in all likelihood, nothing will happen for twenty-four hours, and that thirty-six hours is not an unreasonable amount of time to be in the hospital before baby arrives… So bring entertainment. Diligently following hospital instructions, we arrived for our 18:00 appointment with two days' worth of stuff. We had DVDs and laptops, iPods, books, multiple changes of clothes, toiletries, newborn nappies, first outfits for the little one, a hat to put on him when he was born, baby blankets, and a pillow with the face of a pug that was as ugly as all hell. (On a side note, I am happy to say that the pillow got so drenched in various bodily fluids throughout the birth that it had to go in the bin almost immediately afterwards!) With our stockpile, it was going to take two journeys to the car to move in. We prioritised and agreed that we would take the fun stuff in first and, once we were settled in and the midwives had got things rolling, I would go back for the post-birth essentials.

Our plan worked pretty well – we had our supplies to last us through the night and I scheduled my trip to the car for when my wife went to sleep. But she wasn't sleeping. She had gas and was scared of the impending labour, but mostly complained of gas. She asked the nurse on duty for something to settle her stomach and was seemingly fobbed off, told to go back to bed, and to come back later. This felt really off, given the attentiveness of all the hospital staff so far… As my wife went to the bathroom yet again, the penny lowered (I would say that the penny dropped but it didn't, it was a slow arrival to a conclusion). This was twenty-two hours early… Women had told me, "She'll know when she's in labour!" offensively often… Is it really happening? Is this *it*?

I'd downloaded a contraction timing app, back when we thought I might be timing contractions in preparation to call the number that was highlighted on the front of my wife's birth notes. So I started doing something odd – I started timing my wife's gas. I didn't tell her, not yet, because, if I was wrong, I was actually timing her digestive discomfort, which is a creepy thing to do. But the gas pains became regular, and more intense, and more frequent. This strange activity ended when I was politely asked by my wife why the fuck I was playing on my phone while she was in pain, couldn't sleep, and still didn't know when her labour would start. I responded in the least dramatic way I could… By slowly rotating the phone around to her and telling her that her gas was now four minutes apart (we can laugh about it now).

The next few hours went as the textbooks and the classes had said they would. We'd prepared really well for the labour part, we tried the positions from the birth classes, the massages really helped, and things progressed slowly but they were moving. Until they stopped moving. After an hour of pushing, it became obvious that the baby was stuck. This is where the excitement waned and concern started to set in. I don't want to go into details of every step of the process, but this is where being a birth partner really felt *real*. There were decisions to make, there were people trying to make decisions for us. I joked before the birth at the level of detail that my wife had put into her whole A4 side of birth preferences, but they were a godsend. I had them committed to memory and I am so glad I'd done so. My wife was no longer in a position to make informed decisions, the pain and the exhaustion had set in, she couldn't hear everything that people were asking her or telling her through the pain of the contractions, and I was the one who had to advocate on her behalf. If we hadn't prepared in the way that we had, the rest of the birth would have gone very differently. Now I can't say that the other options would have been *bad*... But what I do know is that our journey left mother and baby both fine, my wife with a birth that she'd wanted, and her gas finally gone.

Mum and Baby were wheeled into a recovery room and everything slowed down. We saw our little boy's face and agreed on his name, my wife had tea and toast, the midwives perched a little woolly hat on top of his ginormous head, and I quickly realised that we didn't have a change of nappies or clothes.

Our son fell asleep. My wife fell asleep. And I went to get the bags from the car.

Birth Journey W

Mother: We were induced on a Wednesday evening – I'd developed gestational diabetes, we'd struggled with conception, and I have a bicornet uterus. Pregnancy had been hard but we were just glad that baby was healthy – that's all that really mattered.

Father: Although my wife was focussed on baby, it was hard seeing her go through pain with sickness throughout the nine months... All the blood tests, all the meetings...

Mother: Following induction, we played a lot of monopoly, did laps of the hospital – walking miles! Twenty-four hours after induction had been started, I then had a pessary inserted, which kick-started the contractions. By this point, I was already shattered – I'd hardly had any sleep being on a bay with three other beds. The midwives on the ward, though amazingly lovely, were low in numbers and overworked, so I had to remind them to monitor me and baby several times as they kept forgetting to do it.

Father: It was hard watching... The fear that something might happen to the baby and, due to previous illness, I had to step in and speak to the midwives about making sure they monitored mum and baby when they were meant to. It was very concerning that we'd been told how important the monitoring was but then it wasn't happening.

Mother: From Friday morning I was told we'd be going through to the delivery suite. This didn't happen. I asked for more than just paracetamol to help with the contractions, but they didn't have anything available besides Pethidine, which I didn't want, seeing as how I was already chundering constantly. They told me to relax as they were capable of delivering on the ward if necessary. My point was, "Well, obviously not, as you don't have gas and air or anything."

Finally, after a lot of pestering and tears as I was just shattered, we got moved to delivery. We were all so tired. My waters were broken... This was probably the worst part as it took a lot of hands up in places where you don't really want them poking around. The gas and air was a lifesaver... Though I was slapped back around as I did manage to pass out on it. Following the breaking of my waters, we did a lot of dealing with the contractions. It got to the point where I needed help, I was just so shattered. Husband was shattered too. I can remember thinking that the waters must have flooded the room, there was so much liquid! I was given an epidural and spent the next few hours power-napping and pushing! It *is* possible to sleep between contractions when you're that tired.

Father: The epidural certainly helped and made mum more comfortable and calmer.

Mother: Unfortunately, baby just did not want to come out, so we were taken to theatre and I was given an episiotomy, and forceps were used to bring him into the world.

It was bizarre having so many people around. But, to be honest, all I cared about was that he was okay. I remember that throughout,

I just kept saying to myself, "As long as he's okay, that's all that matters."

Father: It was amazing and beautiful meeting my little man for the first time properly. After giving birth, my wife had a partial haemorrhage… Though I was confident that we were in the right place, the sight of all of the blood will always stay with me.

Mother: Finally, with baby safe and sound, we managed to get some well-deserved sleep. And lots and lots of cuddles!

The process wasn't easy or as straightforward as we'd all wished it to be but, at the end of the day, the advice given by the midwives and their kindness, as well as that of the other staff, including the lady who went out of her way to try to find me food I could keep down as well as working with the gestational diabetes, was amazing. It's just such a shame they're understaffed and so rushed off their feet.

I think part of me hadn't realised how physically draining and mentally testing giving birth would be. Even once baby was here, not peeing myself was a massive issue and one I've failed to stop on several occasions. But it's all worth it to see him nine months on – learning to walk, babbling to us, and smiling and clapping.

Father: Given all the trials and troubles, it was worth it. It's a shame that those who threw tantrums were the ones that got prioritised and were given priority over couples like us who were trying to calmly get on it. It's obviously a bit of a cultural thing within the hospital – we were advised to kick up a bit of a fuss in order to get through to delivery. At the end of the day though, we have a beautiful baby boy and everyone's healthy and happy.

Birth Journey X

I always thought pregnancy was a joyous experience. I'd been through two pregnancies previously and I knew it was hard but, despite the ups and downs that came with being classed as a "high-risk" pregnancy, I was still grateful that I could grow and carry my babies safely. Adjusting to my new role as Mum wasn't without its difficulties though – after my first child was born, I suffered with postnatal depression and anxiety. I had treatment and support and, before I knew it, I was a working mum with two happy and beautiful children.

But, just when I thought I had life sussed, I was dealt a card that I never expected to face – an unplanned pregnancy.

To understand my birth journey, you need to hear the whole story…

The first few months of my third pregnancy were a rollercoaster of emotions. I wasn't physically or emotionally prepared for another pregnancy. I was excited, I was scared, I was happy, and I was completely outside my comfort zone. I'd accepted with ease the thought of becoming a mother of three, but I could not accept that this would mean another pregnancy and another labour.

I was still on maternity leave when I found out I was pregnant and I was due to return to quite a physical job when I was about 10 weeks pregnant. I wanted to go back to work and I wanted the opportunity to find my identity as a working mum. I don't think I really made a conscious decision not to tell anyone about my pregnancy but, before I knew it, only a handful of very close family and friends knew. In hindsight, this is probably where my anxiety started to grow. I was already attending frequent medical appointments because of pre-existing medical conditions and I was diagnosed very early on with gestational diabetes. Already this pregnancy was following the same trajectory as my previous two, except now I was juggling two young children, a full-time job, all whilst trying to find time to attend medical appointments without anyone finding out.

As the weeks went by, I became more anxious about concealing my pregnancy at work. Every time I tried to talk about it, I found that I could never get the words out. Instead of opening up, I kept convincing myself to have just one more week of "normality" before everything changed for good. By keeping it to myself, I found I had an environment where I could forget the worries that came with this pregnancy. I was 23 weeks pregnant when I finally opened up and, even then, this was only out of necessity – I was approached by a colleague who asked me outright if I was pregnant again – and I realised that I could no longer deny my ever-growing bump.

After this, my mental health noticeably declined. I was tired all the time and my mood was low. My immune system was taking a battering from the endless coughs and colds that kept circulating through our household and I started avoiding friends. I had the energy to look after my children and go to work; everything else was placed on the backburner. I recognised at this stage that I wasn't very well and I saw my GP who gave me wonderful help and support. Unfortunately, I was not prepared for the crushing depression and anxiety that came next.

For the last three months of my pregnancy I was unrecognisable to myself and to my husband. Most days I didn't want to get out of bed, let alone leave the house. I did everything I could to stay at home in the security of my own four walls. I started missing hospital appointments. Initially, I made excuses as to why I could not attend but soon, I just gave up contacting anyone. I was unable to look after my own health and I was not able to manage the medication I needed to take to keep my baby safe. I knew I was harming myself and I knew I was harming my unborn baby, but I felt paralysed by the black cloud I had over me. I convinced myself that I didn't deserve this beautiful baby I was carrying.

When I had better days, I was able to recognise that something was wrong. I know that this is what saved me because, on those days, I told anyone who would listen that I needed help. I begged for help. Unfortunately for me, my local maternity unit did not have a midwife who specialised in mental health. Eventually, over concerns that my physical health was declining, I was admitted for an induction two days earlier than planned.

By this stage, I wasn't sure I had even bonded with my baby. I had convinced myself that my baby needed a better mum. I was terrified of how I would manage. My delivery was more complicated than my previous two deliveries. It was the middle of the night when I went into active labour. I had been told that they were withholding the next stage of the induction and would continue the process in the morning, but my body had a mind of its own and suddenly the "plan" was a distant memory. I was exhausted.

My baby was not in the ideal position and it was harder to push. With lots of help, I eventually delivered a beautiful baby boy. I should have been euphoric when my baby was handed straight to me but instead, I looked down at a silent and still baby. I panicked.

I begged the midwife to take him back, I begged them to do something, the emergency buzzer was pressed, and the room filled with people. The cord had become wrapped around his neck and he wasn't breathing by himself. What happened next is now a blur. They rushed him away and started helping him with his breathing. After a few minutes, he started breathing for himself but, to me, it felt like a lifetime.

You never know how you will react or feel when put into that situation. My baby was given back to me when he was breathing but I was numb by that stage. I still hadn't delivered my placenta and it was stuck. I was bleeding heavily. I felt as though I wanted to give up. At the time, I remember feeling so ashamed because I had asked them to take my baby away from me… I couldn't even hold my own baby. I had nothing left to give and I was still surrounded by midwives and doctors. The theatre was prepped, but just as the decision was made to take me to theatre, my placenta delivered.

For the next hour, I could not bring myself to hold my baby. He lay in the cot next to my bed and I cried. I blamed myself entirely. After a while, I went to sleep. I was scared to wake up again. But when I did wake up, the fog had started to lift. Something changed and I suddenly didn't want to let my baby go. I can't say that I recovered instantly but, in that moment, I was able to experience joy again.

My worry was that I would never bond with my son, but I had nothing to worry about because I've got the happiest baby boy who loves and adores me, his dad, and his siblings unconditionally. He has completed our family and brought us all closer. I am still recovering, but I am recovering with three wonderful children by my side. I still have periods where I feel low and I do sometimes feel anxious, but I know now that it's okay to not be okay. More importantly, I know it's good to talk and I know it's good to listen.

Birth Journey Y

Pick one moment from your labour and describe how you felt.

I'd been in labour since Friday evening. I made the typical trip to hospital in the early hours to be told that I was only 2cm dilated and sent back home with, "It could be days," rolling round my head. Contractions were very strong all morning and, by early afternoon, I was not finding the TENS machine helpful. I was, quite frankly, knackered, so my partner suggested I have a bath. I got in, put a hypnobirthing track on my phone, and lay back to relax. The water felt amazing – what they say about that is so true! The contractions didn't stop but I was able to tune out and rest up a bit in the water. It was while I was still in the water (and, I think, probably as a consequence of chilling out and letting go a bit) that my contractions started to change and I felt the urge to push. It felt like my body had taken over and I wasn't in control. The pressure was intense and I felt like I was failing to hold back… From my body pushing for me or from making weird groaning noises. Somehow the noises helped to deal with the pain. It was strange and a bit scary… And it was then that I knew it was time to get back on the phone to the maternity unit and say that we were on our way.

Describe two contrasting moments from your labour.

We spent ages in early labour holed up together in the living room, trying to bounce it out on the ball, doing hip circles on all fours, figuring out how the TENS machine worked, and then downloading an app to time contractions. I wanted something distracting but not demanding to help pass the time, so we watched *so* many episodes of vintage *Grand Designs*. My partner and I felt like such a team. It was lovely to feel so close and together, and like the whole world (apart from nineties' building projects!) didn't exist.

When we finally got to hospital it turned out I was ready to push. The position I found most comfortable was lying on the bed on my back (I know, I know... The absolute worst position for *actually* getting a baby out but that's what I wanted) with my face in my partner's stomach and arms around his torso. Thinking about it, I don't really understand how I got in that position but, during contractions I turned my face into him and somehow that made me feel nice. I really needed him and, although I know he thinks he was a bit of a spare part, he was definitely integral to me getting through it.

How did you feel when labour began?

I went into labour at 39 weeks, so I was a bit caught out after hearing that all first babies are late(!) I was kind of excited but really daunted too... And also peeved that I hadn't had time to chill out beforehand because I'd only finished work three days earlier. I had box sets lined up! I'd also planned to do a couple of days of practical things (like batch cooking) to get over my guilt at finishing work while my partner still had to go... Before just putting my feet up and chilling. In the end, I only did the practical stuff and none of the relaxation, and it was scary thinking, "This is it!" as the rest of my life spiralled away in front of me, all different and new... It felt a lot like an ending.

Did your experience influence your thoughts about birthing future children?

I have a few regrets about my labour experience… I ended up doing most of it alone at home with two paracetamol and I felt cheated out of my hopes for a birth pool and gas and air. I think, probably, that that was generally a good thing and I'm so lucky I didn't need any more intense help or have to be in a consultant-led ward. Although I do hold such a long time contracting and such a drawn-out period of pain responsible for such a long pushing stage – it took hours. In the end, my contractions started disappearing and I couldn't push the baby all the way out, so had an episiotomy. Anyway, after all that, I immediately thought, "Next time I will know what to do, know when it feels like the right time to go to hospital, get my pool, not be so tired, not need the cut, etc." I feel competitive with myself that I'll do a much better job next time.

How did you feel about your interventions?

I had an episiotomy after the baby's head was on the cusp of coming out for what seemed like, and might actually have been, hours. I really didn't want this. When I first got to hospital and talked through my birth preferences with my midwife, the only thing I said was, "I don't want a cut." I tried and tried to get him out without one and the midwives supported me with that, bringing in extra encouragement, getting my partner to really help me on… But, in the end, they were concerned about the baby's heart rate and I was worried because my contractions were much less intense and I wanted to avoid anything more drastic, so I agreed to it. I feel disappointed really about it and I had issues with the healing, which felt scary and horrible at the time. My regular midwife, who came out to look after me at home, said she sees far more issues with episiotomies healing than with tearing, which I wasn't aware of before. I had done some perineal massage before labour but definitely not as much as I could have done… So next time I'll certainly apply myself to that better!

Did your birth experience match your birth preferences or expectations? Did you consider yourself prepared for labour?

Yes and no. I wanted to labour in the midwife-led unit and that's where I went… But I did have my heart set on using a pool. By the time we'd gone back into hospital and I was examined, I was 9cm dilated and ready to push, and I didn't feel like I wanted to do that in the pool.

Labour lasted such a long time and I really wish I'd been better rested beforehand… But I'd been waking up very early and having trouble getting comfortable enough to sleep for weeks, so that was maybe beyond my control.

What I think I wasn't really prepared for was all the blood and the sort of visceral nature of the whole thing, which is kind of obvious, but I just hadn't experienced anything like it before. I was also really unprepared to actually *look after* the baby once he arrived. I didn't know what to do. Despite all the books, I felt a bit shell-shocked and wired and out of my depth. But I think regardless of how much I'd prepared, I still would have felt that way.

How supportive was your birth partner?

My birth partner was amazing… Apart from having almost run out of petrol entirely on the drive to the hospital (something which he sensibly only told me later on). I feel like we were a real team and that was good.

Describe what labour felt like.

It's hard to remember it properly, looking back… I feel like I'm looking back on the memory through fog or something. I know it bloody hurt! At home I used a TENS machine, which was good but probably more as a distraction. I liked having something to do and fiddling with the levels did that!

I did prenatal yoga classes and our instructor suggested useful positions for labour. Being on all fours and circling hips was good, as was sitting on the ball and circling or bouncing, and kneeling by the bed and leaning on it with my top half. The time between coming back home from hospital the first time and going back again (probably between about 07:00 and 16:00) is a bit of a blur to recollect. I moved around the house between beds and sofas, trying to get comfortable, and basically nowhere did the job for long. I remember that lying down in between contractions was nice but I couldn't stay lying down *during* contractions. I took a couple of paracetamols that probably did something, but I couldn't tell you what!

When I got into hospital (finally), I used gas and air, which again I think was partially good because it felt like I was doing something about the pain. It didn't take the pain away totally but maybe made it feel a bit fuzzier, less distinct.

Describe the moment when you met your baby.

I think the overriding feeling was confusion. The whole process took so long and then suddenly was all over with a gush and there he was and I was being stitched up. Very bizarre. I felt relief that it was done and that he'd arrived. But it took a while for me to experience the warm feelings and to get excited about his tiny hands and feet and little movements.

Birth Journey Z

It might sound strange, but I remember having this *feeling* before I went into labour. I went to bed that night with the usual routine – faffing with the pregnancy pillow until I found the least uncomfortable position and singing to my baby bump to wish him goodnight. An unusual feeling came over me that's hard to put into words... It was a sort of peaceful feeling, a readiness that I hadn't ever felt before. Weird, hey? Within half an hour, just after 22:00, I was awake again, in labour. I was one of the 1 in 10 women whose labour starts with her waters breaking. I remember waking up very suddenly, stumbling to the bathroom in the dark, and saying to my husband, "Either I've just wet myself, or I'm in labour."

"Shit," we both thought. "This is it!"

I had to *actually* give birth to an *actual* baby. I was a little excited but, at this point, primarily somewhat terrified.

Now, when my waters broke it was the full shebang. I belonged in the "gushing" category (something about that choice of word makes me feel a bit gross!) It went on for what felt like an hour and made it through various pairs of pyjama bottoms. We rang the midwife-led unit when my waters first broke and were advised about things we needed to look out for that could indicate a problem. Otherwise, we just needed to sit tight at home and wait until my contractions were three minutes apart.

In our antenatal classes we'd been told that during the early stages of labour you're best to go to bed and try to sleep... "You'll need any rest you can get!" So, when my waters finally stopped soaking everything in sight, I got back into bed. Well, I don't know if it was because my labour had started with my waters breaking (I have heard that this can make the first contractions more painful) but how anyone could ever sleep through contractions is an absolute mystery to me! There's something about your whole body being taken over by intense pain (for what, in reality, is probably less than a minute but, at the time, feels like an age) that isn't exactly conducive to sleep! So, instead of sleeping, I sent my husband back to bed while I went downstairs; he was the one who would have to drive me to hospital when the time came.

For the next three-four hours I tried to distract myself with TV, use some of the positions I'd learnt in my pregnancy yoga class (they definitely did provide a bit of pain relief), and attempted "mindful breathing" through each contraction. I was supported by my furry birth partner, my springer spaniel, through those first few hours, and I think he might have had the most calming effect out of everything I tried at home. I remember watching countless episodes of *Unbreakable Kimmy Schmidt* on Netflix… Who knows why, I don't even like it that much! I guess I just needed something that I could tune out of for a minute at a time and not miss much of the plot!

By about 03:00, I was aware that my contractions were getting really strong; I was completely tuning out during each one. I woke my husband and he rang the midwifery unit. Between contractions I explained to him that some were five minutes apart, but others were only two and a half or three minutes apart. I still remember that they asked to speak with me and my husband tried to give me the phone mid-contraction. All I could manage was to shake my head.

"Is this your first baby?" we were asked. "Oh no, everything's fine. Just stay at home and don't come in until your contractions are *consistently* three minutes apart."

After almost another hour, I'd had enough. They kept telling us to stay at home, but I felt certain it was time to go to the hospital… So I figured that the best thing I could say to them over the phone (so that they'd let me come in) was to tell them that I needed more pain relief. If I asked for extra pain relief, they couldn't really refuse me. I'm so glad I trusted my instincts and didn't listen to the advice to wait for consistency… My contractions never did become consistently close together.

We arrived at the midwifery unit at 05:00 after a very stressful drive for my husband, waited and rang the bell for what felt like forever, were taken to a room, and then almost immediately left. This moment was one of the lowest for me – I had no idea what I was doing, I was terrified of giving birth, the pain was getting worse, and we were alone. The midwife returned briefly to bring gas and air, and to tell me very firmly to stop shouting because "that won't help anything". I was scared and upset, and my husband could see it, so he asked (probably not in the politest way) for her to stay with me. We got a very defensive (frankly arsy) response: "We're very busy tonight, I can't just stay here." She returned later to check dilation (7cm) and to bring some Diamorphine that I'd wanted about an hour ago but now no longer wanted (the gas and air was finally starting to kick in… Besides, Diamorphine wasn't in The All-Important Birth Plan!) I wish I'd felt more empowered to complain and ask for another midwife… I think I'd definitely do that if I were to have another baby.

My husband and I were both relieved at 07:30 when the shifts changed over. We were suddenly blessed with an absolute angel of a midwife who didn't leave my side for the rest of labour.

At some point that I can't quite remember, I was given the first dose of IV antibiotics (now this *was* in The All-Important Birth Plan as I'd tested positive for Group B streptococcus early on in pregnancy).

The next five and a half hours are a bit of a blur. What I do remember is that my husband was an absolute rock, pandering to my every demand, and providing calm, steady encouragement that I could do this. I remember getting the sensation to push quite soon after the new midwife came on shift and being encouraged to push if I felt like I should. Well, as I eventually discovered a few hours later, when the midwife was "up close and personal" and looking at my baby's hair poking through, I wasn't actually pushing in the most effective way. Wish I'd known that before wasting those hours exhausting myself without getting very far! I remember moving between positions – standing, kneeling, crouching – but eventually my feet were numb and I was spent. By 10:00, I was 10cm dilated and my midwife encouraged me to spend some time lying on the bed (not in The All-Important but oh, what a relief!)

Then we hit another trough… Although one that I now look back on with humour! I had the urge to wee. The midwife said that this might actually help get baby "round the bend"… But I just couldn't go. So I ended up sitting on the toilet, legs wide open, pushing along with my contractions, crying, "I can't do it!", insisting that I couldn't possibly move anywhere else, and having to be hauled off by my midwife and husband so that Baby wouldn't be welcomed into the world in a toilet bowl. I was catheterised

(something that I previously would have dreaded but frankly this just felt like a minor inconvenience compared to the contractions!)

For almost three hours the midwife and my husband kept looking at my vagina – they could see Baby's head, he was "nearly there!" At one point I was even shown what was going on using a strategically positioned mirror, which just freaked me out! By 12:30, after several hours of pushing, it was decided that baby was not, in fact, "nearly there" enough; we would have to go to another room for an assisted ventouse delivery. *Definitely* not in The All-Important but I was so happy! Knowing that I didn't have to keep vainly trying to get him out and that I'd meet him soon was a great reassurance… The end was in sight!

The team who delivered our baby were amazing, so professional. I was set up in stirrups, they came in, introduced themselves and their roles, and talked me through everything they were doing. I did not object to the episiotomy – whatever it took to get my baby out! My husband kept one hand on mine and the other on the oxygen mask throughout. Then, after a few final big pushes, I suddenly heard the cry of my little baby. Before I knew it, he was there on my chest, screaming his cone-shaped head off. My husband shed a tear, but I didn't cry. The overriding feeling at that point was relief – relief that Baby was okay, relief that labour was almost over.

I felt too exhausted to even consider trying to deliver the placenta myself, so I asked for Syntocinon (guess what? Also not in The All-Important). I remember the placenta was delivered without issue… But then the doctor very calmly informed me and the other staff that I was losing more blood (a postpartum haemorrhage). Luckily, I was in the best place for the situation in hand and, with a few injections, the bleeding stopped (I lost an estimated 800ml in total). Throughout all this I remained very calm; I had my baby on my chest, I was in safe hands, people were doing what they needed to do. I think this part was a lot more distressing for my husband, who had an entirely different vantage point and was acutely aware of just how much 800ml of blood really is.

After the doctors had stitched me up and were happy that all was well, I was wheeled back round to the previous room. Suddenly, I became clearly focussed on my husband carrying our tiny baby in his arms – a proud, exhausted, and emotional new father who had, if anything, just played the more emotionally draining role out the two of us. We were finally given some time alone with our baby… Lovely, slightly terrifying… I'm still not sure I quite believed it was real. I was exhausted, relieved, and in a lot of pain (I only moved from the bed when I absolutely had to). I was happy to be with my baby, but I didn't have that overwhelming feeling of love that some people describe. That feeling took time. I think I might have been in shock, a bit like a rabbit in the headlights, as the realisation dawned that I was responsible for keeping this tiny little person safe.

I remember saying to my husband, "I'm never doing this again. If I change my mind, remind me of this." Now *that* feeling *has* definitely changed. I won't say that it changed in a week, or even in two weeks, but it did change. Now I look back and can say that I would do it all again. We're so lucky to be parents and my son is such a gift. He's changed our lives in ways we could have never imagined and that is why I'd do it again… Because all the pain and fear and exhaustion simply pale in comparison to the pride and joy that he has brought us.

Afterword

This book is clearly not representative of all birth experiences – C-sections are underrepresented, only supportive birth partners are described, every mother-to-be could access an appropriate medical facility when one was needed, and all stories end with a living mother and baby, for example. This collection is also, by nature, reflective. Varying amounts of time have passed since these births occurred and their stories told – for some writers it was merely weeks but, for others, it was decades. Time is downright devilish for changing our perspective and perception of events, how they felt, and how they made us feel. And let's not forget the warping, shape-shifting powers of those juicy postnatal hormones!

Nevertheless, these birth journeys have been written with the honest intention of exploring labour's highs, lows, and everything in-betweens. Without considering what is or isn't appropriate to share. Without knowing who's reading and their experience of, preconceptions about, and attitudes towards birth and all its baggage. The stark openness of these birth journeys is, I believe, both refreshing and vital, especially when placed against today's backdrop of parent shaming and judgement.

All contributors tried their very best to describe an intricate, dense, and knotty ball of emotions that is tricky to tease apart. The need for the women in labour to feel in control of and in tune with what was happening to their bodies, to make decisions that were informed (even when there was only one decision that could safely be made), and for the momentous nature of these experiences to be taken seriously simply leaps off these pages. Many writers detailed the tremendous pressure under which NHS staff were operating. For many contributors, gauging when or waiting to be invited to travel to hospital was a key emotional milestone. Many explained how fatigue felt as brutal as the pain. For some, a small, fleeting action entirely re-routed their birth journey – a whisper, passing comment, supportive touch, quick glance – for better or for worse. Some mothers betrayed feeling a pressure, a burden to "succeed". For these women, at some point in pregnancy (or even beforehand), a picture – *The Perfect Birth* – was painted. But one woman's dream birth – a drug-free water birth at home – could be the nightmare of a mother-to-be who's booked in for her elective C-section (and vice versa). If a birth journey does not progress as planned, the emotional fallout for parents can be (and often is) devastating. And all parents who wrote or spoke for this book found previously untapped strengths when they believed that their physical, mental, and emotional reserves had been sucked bone dry.

I laid out this collection's aims in the introduction – to provide a kaleidoscopic snapshot of the childbirth experience, to allow parents to share their birth stories uninterrupted, and to begin forging a language of childbirth. Working towards these aims has revealed our next step – we need to do better, as individuals and as a society, for labouring women and their families. Our responsibility now is to move the conversation beyond pain and pain relief as badges of honour, beyond what constitutes a "natural" birthing experience, beyond birth plans and preferences, and to talk about what it really feels like to birth a child into the world and to respect the emotions that this particular journey into parenthood entails. We can start by sharing our birth stories as far and as wide as they'll go, freeing them to embark on their own illuminating, reassuring, informative, and empowering journeys, and by actively listening to those that we hear and acknowledging how they make us feel. Because, one way or another, our babies will be birthed. And how we feel about these journeys in the moment, and for years to come, is really rather important.

Glossary

I have absolutely no professional medical experience or training; the following definitions are nothing more than a combination of my own research and experience. They are provided solely to help someone with no prior knowledge of pregnancy and childbirth understand the birth journeys told in this collection.

Anti-D injection: Medication that can prevent Rhesus disease.

Amniotic fluid: Fluid filling the amniotic sac inside a woman's womb where the unborn baby develops and grows.

Bicornet uterus: A uterus with a deep indentation at the top.

Birth plan / Birth preferences: A written document describing what a woman would like to happen during labour and delivery.

Braxton Hicks: Also called "practice contractions". When the woman's abdominal muscles tighten but the cervix does not dilate.

Breech: When a baby's buttocks or legs are nearest the cervix instead of his/her head.

Caesarean / C-section: Surgical operation to deliver a baby by cutting through the wall of the mother's abdomen.

Cord blood banking: Donating blood taken from the placenta and umbilical cord after the birth of a baby as it is rich in blood stem cells.

Crowning: When the head of the baby is passing through the vaginal opening.

Dilation: When the cervix gradually opens so the baby can exit the womb.

Due date: The estimated day when parents can expect to meet their baby. A pregnancy normally lasts between 37 and 42 weeks.

Entonox: See **Gas and air**.

Epidural: Local anaesthetic injected in the spine for pain relief.

Episiotomy: A cut made in the area between the vagina and anus during childbirth, widening the vaginal opening so the baby can pass through more easily.

External cephalic version: When a healthcare professional tries to turn a breech baby into a head-down position by applying pressure on the mother's abdomen.

Forceps: Smooth metal instruments resembling tongs that are used to pull the baby out as the mother pushes with a contraction.

Full term: A pregnancy lasting between 37 and 42 weeks.

Gas and air: A mixture of oxygen and nitrous oxide gas (Entonox) used for pain relief in labour.

Gestational diabetes: High blood sugar that develops during pregnancy and usually disappears after the baby's birth.

Hospital bag: A bag packed with all the supplies a family might need during labour and for the first few hours or days after the baby's birth.

Hyperemesis gravidarum: Excessive nausea and vomiting in pregnancy.

Hypnobirthing: A self-help method to manage pain and anxiety during childbirth that involves therapeutic relaxation techniques, such as different breathing patterns and visualisations.

Induction: A labour started artificially in hospital.

IUS: Intrauterine system. A small T-shaped plastic contraceptive device that is inserted into a woman's womb.

Meconium: The first black tarry stool from a newborn baby.

Mucous plug: "Seals" the cervix during pregnancy and comes away during or close to the start of labour. Acts as a barrier to protect the baby from bacteria.

NCT: National Childbirth Trust. A charity who support parents through birth and early parenthood. Expectant parents can pay to attend classes hosted by NCT to learn about pregnancy, birth, and early parenthood, and to meet local parents expecting babies at a similar time.

NICU: Neonatal Intensive Care Unit.

Perineum: The area between the vaginal opening and the anus.

Pethidine: A drug injected to help relieve pain.

PICU: Paediatric Intensive Care Unit.

Placenta: The organ attached to the mother's womb lining during pregnancy. The placenta keeps the baby's blood supply separate from the mother's but provides a link between the two; this means it can carry out functions that the unborn baby cannot.

Post-term / Prolonged / Overdue: A pregnancy lasting longer than 42 weeks.

Preeclampsia: A condition affecting some pregnant women. It's marked by high blood pressure and a high level of protein in their urine.

Preterm / Premature: A pregnancy lasting less than 37 weeks.

Rhesus negative / positive: A blood test can show if a mother's blood type is rhesus negative or positive. If a mother is rhesus negative and she has a rhesus positive baby, the baby's blood can enter her bloodstream. Her immune system can then develop antibodies against it that then attack the baby's red blood cells.

Skin-to-skin: Holding baby naked or wearing only a nappy against parent's skin.

Spinal block: Anaesthetic injected near the spinal cord to block pain.

Stages of labour: Labour consists of three stages:
   First stage: Contracting to dilate the cervix. Labour is established when the cervix has dilated to more than 3cm and regular contractions are opening the cervix. The first stage ends when the cervix is 10cm dilated.
   Second stage: Also called "the pushing phase". From when the cervix is fully dilated until the birth of the baby.
   Third stage: Delivering the placenta after the baby is born.

Stretch and sweep / Sweep: A midwife or doctor "sweeps" a finger around the mother's cervix to separate the amniotic sac's membranes from the cervix. This separation releases hormones that may then kick-start the woman's labour.

TENS machine: A device delivering transcutaneous electrical nerve stimulation. Electrodes are taped onto the woman's back that are connected by wires to a small battery-powered stimulator. The woman can then give herself small safe amounts of current through the electrodes as a form of pain relief.

Transition: Progressing from the first stage of labour to the second. Often described as the most intense and challenging part of labour.

Umbilical cord: A cord connecting the baby in the womb to its mother.

Ventouse: A cup-shaped suction device that can be attached to the baby's head. It helps to pull the baby out as the mother pushes during a contraction.

Call for Contributors, or Coming Soon

The next volume of *An A-Z of Real Parenthood Journeys* will focus on infant feeding – by boobs, bottles, and both. If you have a story to share, please e-mail Rosemari Bainbridge – realbirthjourneys@gmail.com.

46327521R00094

Printed in Poland
by Amazon Fulfillment
Poland Sp. z o.o., Wrocław